Philosophy of Nursing

Also by Steven D. Edwards

Philosophical Issues in Nursing (1998)
Nursing Ethics: A Principle-Based Approach (1996)
Externalism in the Philosophy of Mind (1994)
Relativism, Conceptual Schemes and Categorial Frameworks (1990)

Philosophy of Nursing
An Introduction

Steven D. Edwards
RMN, BA(Hons), MPhil, PhD

palgrave

First published 2001 by
PALGRAVE
Houndmills, Basingstoke, Hampshire RG21 6XS and
175 Fifth Avenue, New York, N.Y. 10010
Companies and representatives throughout the world

PALGRAVE is the new global academic imprint of
St. Martin's Press LLC Scholarly and Reference Division and
Palgrave Publishers Ltd (formerly Macmillan Press Ltd).

ISBN 0–333–74991–X paperback

This book is printed on paper suitable for recycling and
made from fully managed and sustained forest sources.

A catalogue record for this book is available
from the British Library.

Editing and origination by
Aardvark Editorial, Mendham, Suffolk

10 9   8   7   6   5   4   3   2   1
10 09 08 07 06 05 04 03 02 01

Printed in Great Britain by
Creative Print & Design (Wales), Ebbw Vale

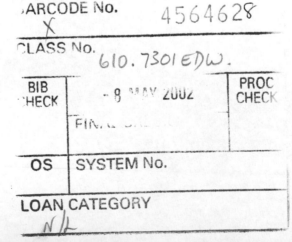

For JL, RL & JL

Contents

Acknowledgements   ix

Introduction   1

1   The nature of philosophy of nursing   3
    Historical matters   3
    Philosophical enquiry   6
    Philosophy of nursing   14
    The conceptual location of philosophy of nursing   18

2   Nursing knowledge (i): propositional and practical   21
    Defining propositional knowledge   21
    Practical knowledge   31

3   Nursing knowledge (ii): Carper and Benner on knowledge   40
    Carper's 'Fundamental Patterns of Knowing in Nursing'
        (1978) (FPKN)   40
    Benner on knowledge: (a) novice/expert; (b) intuition;
        (c) propositional and practical knowing   49
    What is nursing knowledge?   60
    Conclusion   65

4   Nursing the person (i): ontology   67
    Introduction   67
    Four accounts of the person   72
    Evaluation   84

5   Nursing the person (ii): the individual person as a narrative   87
    A narrative conception of the person   87
    Nursing and the narrative view of the person   93
    Conclusions   105

6   Care in nursing (i): intentional care   109
    Intentional care   109
    Noddings and care   114
    Care, emotion and two problems   119
    Conclusion   122

7   **Care in nursing (ii): ontological care**   124
     Ontological care   124
     Intentional care in nursing revisited   131
     Summary   134

8   **The nature of nursing (i): nursing as a science**   136
     Clarifying the claim that nursing is a science   136
     Positivism   142
     Interpretivism   145
     Realism   150
     Conclusion   155

9   **The nature of nursing (ii): nursing as art or practice**   157
     Nursing as an art   157
     Nursing as a practice   164
     Conclusion   172

10   **The prospects for a theory of nursing**   175
     Preamble   175
     Dickoff and James on theory   177
     Generalisations and narratives   181
     Two further problems   185

Conclusion   192

Glossary   195

Notes   197

Bibliography   200

Index   208

Acknowledgements

In writing this book I have been fortunate enough to work in an environment where philosophy of nursing is taken seriously. So it has been possible to discuss the ideas explored within the book with many students and colleagues. It is not possible to mention all those who have helped my thinking in the area of philosophy of nursing, but I owe very considerable debts of gratitude to Louise de Raeve, Paul Wainwright, Keith Cash, Diana Moore, David Greaves, John Paley and Martyn Evans. Particular thanks are due to John Paley. He was kind enough to read an earlier version of this book and to make many helpful comments and criticisms which have enabled me to improve its content considerably. Needless to add, remaining errors are my sole responsibility.

Finally, I would like to thank the editors and publishers of *Nursing Ethics* and the *Journal of Advanced Nursing* for their permission to include extracts from two papers published in these journals. The papers are: 'The art of nursing', *Nursing Ethics* **5**(5), 393–400, 1998; and 'Benner and Wrubel on caring', *Journal of Advanced Nursing* **31**(1), 2001.

STEVEN EDWARDS
Senior Lecturer
Centre for Philosophy and Health Care
University of Wales, Swansea

Introduction

The aim of this book is to provide an introduction to some of the main areas of enquiry within the topic of philosophy of nursing. It is evident that philosophy modules are now included in many courses for nurses, especially at postgraduate level. This book is written with such courses in mind. Indeed it is based on the teaching sessions I have contributed to some of them. It is hoped that the book will be helpful both to those who study philosophy within the nursing context and to those who teach it. For although there are many such courses, there are few books available which attempt a systematic introduction to the subject of philosophy of nursing.

Chapter 1 provides a general outline of the nature of both philosophical enquiry and philosophy of nursing. Philosophical enquiry is divided up, as is customary, into the areas of epistemology, ontology, value-enquiry and logic. Subsequent discussion in the book follows this ordering, roughly speaking.

Chapters 2 and 3 centre on epistemology. Our concern here lies with the question of the nature of knowledge, the distinction (if any) between propositional and practical knowledge, and the idea of intuition as a source of knowledge. Landmark contributions to these issues by Carper (1978) and Benner (1984) are each subjected to critical scrutiny. A position is arrived at in which, in the realms of both propositional and practical knowledge, knowledge should be regarded as revisable. In the light of this it is proposed that the appropriate 'attitude' of knowers towards what they 'know' is one of *modesty*. Also, the view that propositional and practical knowledge differ in kind is supported. Given acceptance of these conclusions concerning knowledge it follows that any credible account of nursing must respect them.

We move in Chapters 4 and 5 to look at a second main area of philosophical enquiry, ontology. Our focus here lies on the person. In Chapter 4 we try to describe an ontology of persons in general such that they are beings with both mental and physical properties (for example mental properties such as thoughts and feelings; and physical properties such as height and weight). This conclusion is reached following discussion of its main rivals. Of course the conclusion does not explain how individual persons differ from one another. To articulate this distinction we appeal to a *narrative* conception of the person. As will be seen, this is a complex idea but is set out by reference to the notions of a self-conception and a self-project. The claim is that a narrative is the description of the pursuance of a self-project. A self-project, as will be seen, can be understood to be driven by a self-conception. We will see how crucial this view of the individual person is to the nursing context. As with the conclusions generated by our discussion of knowledge, accep-

1

tance of our conclusions concerning persons carries the consequence that a credible account of nursing must respect them.

Chapters 6 and 7 focus on the topic of care and, to a limited extent, on the third area of philosophy, value-enquiry. For obvious reasons the topic of care has received much discussion within nursing literature, in particular in relation to the moral dimension of nursing. However, our focus differs slightly. Chapter 6 is most closely related to the explication of care as it contributes to the bringing about of the ends of nursing as these are usually understood. Thus, it focuses on the idea of caring actions, and we try to identify defining characteristics of these. Chapter 7 discusses what is termed *ontological* care. Here we try to clear up some common ambiguities surrounding the idea of care, and to show how the performance of caring acts in nursing relates to the idea of *ontological* care. As will be seen, awareness of care in the ontological sense is presupposed in the idea of intentional care, and the idea of intentional care can be explained by reference to the vulnerability of humans, to their capacity to experience pain and suffering. The very intelligibility of nursing rests upon this aspect of what it is to be human. We will see also that a nurse's capacity to give intentional care is enhanced by appreciation of a further central feature of human existence, termed here 'identity-constituting care'.

We then turn to discuss the nature of nursing. It would be nice, for the sake of neatness, if we could describe this as a discussion within the fourth area of philosophy, logic. However, doing this would require indecent contortions with the sense of this latter term. We consider the question of whether nursing is a science, an art or a practice. On the grounds of the richness of the latter, and the inappropriateness of the other two we opt for the view of nursing as a practice. This, as will be seen, is a notion rich enough to accommodate the nature of knowledge in nursing, that of the person in nursing, and the moral dimension of nursing. Thus it is a notion rich enough to accommodate our findings in epistemology, ontology and value-enquiry.

But, there proves to be a problem. The idea of a practice requires a 'unity' which is threatened by certain of our findings. Specifically, the narrative conception of the person favoured here calls into serious question the possibility of generalisations within nursing. For if patients are all to be treated individually, according to their various narratives, then how can we make generalisations concerning how best to care for them? Thus the unity characteristic of practices seems placed in jeopardy. However, via a focus on the idea of a theory of nursing, Chapter 10 argues that the 'unity requirement' can be met and so nursing can be understood as a practice. It is one in which means and ends are rationally related.

It should be added, finally, that many of the discussions within this book are of equal relevance to medicine, and so can be considered within the context of philosophy of medicine. I have resisted the temptation as far as possible to make any such links explicit, but it is worth signalling here that they can be made without too much effort.

1 The nature of philosophy of nursing

This chapter will begin with a brief historical overview of appeals to philosophy in nursing. We then turn to look at the nature of philosophical enquiry, its distinctive character, main areas, and tools. Following this we look more specifically at philosophy of nursing, its definition, and its main strands. Lastly, we also consider the place of philosophy of nursing within philosophy.

Historical matters

It is reported that Florence Nightingale (1820–1910) received some philosophical education from her father (Marriner-Tomey, 1994, p. 73), and that she engaged in correspondence of a philosophical nature with both Benjamin Jowett and J.S. Mill (Quinn and Prest, 1987).

She is described by Marriner-Tomey as having propounded a specific 'philosophy of nursing' (Marriner-Tomey, 1994, p. 74) and as having a 'nursing philosophy' (ibid.). Roughly, what is meant by philosophy in these last two senses is a general view of nursing: a view of the proper ends of nursing, and the means by which these ends can be brought about. Evidently, Nightingale considered the ends of nursing to consist in the prevention of disease, or its alleviation (*Notes on Nursing*, 1957, p. v). In her view, the means by which these ends can be brought about centre on the importance of ventilation, warmth, nutrition, cleanliness, and light (see *Notes on Nursing*).

It is not important for our present purposes to fill in the details of Nightingale's view. What is noteworthy is the description of her view of nursing as involving the proposal of a *philosophy of nursing*. Indeed, Marriner-Tomey identifies several other eminent nurse scholars as having set out *philosophies* of nursing; these include Virginia Henderson, Ernestine Weidenbach, and Patricia Benner. Marriner-Tomey's justification for describing the views of these scholars as philosophies appears to be that such scholars have the kind of broad vision of nursing in terms of its ends and means which is present in Nightingale's work.

However, there is a sense of the term 'philosophy' which is importantly different from that just described, a sense which we might term its academic sense – one which concerns its use in academic philosophy as practised within philosophy departments in educational institutions and academic publications. This activity differs markedly from the development of general views of nursing, from the development of 'philosophies' in Marriner-Tomey's sense.

3

Moreover, it is an activity in which nursing scholars over the past 40 years or so have taken an increasing interest.

This increase in interest has taken various forms. Most innocuously it has been signalled by the references to philosophical works by nurse scholars. For example, Rogers (1970), Orem (1971) and Roy (1976) published texts on their respective theories of nursing which include references to the works of philosophers. More conspicuously, the increase in interest in philosophy has been manifested in the active involvement of philosophers in nursing scholarship. Famously, this occurred with the work of Dickoff and James (1968); but also has included figures such as J.R. Scudder (for example Bishop and Scudder, 1991), S. Spicker (1980) and A. MacIntyre (1983).

A further level of involvement has been signalled by attempts to ground approaches to nursing on the work of specific philosophers. This is done explicitly by Benner (1984), who invokes the work of Heidegger (1962) and Dreyfus and Dreyfus (1980); and Benner and Wrubel (1989), who base their account of the primacy of caring on the work of Heidegger, Merleau-Ponty (1962), Dreyfus (1991) and Taylor (1985). Also, Parse makes an explicit claim that her own theory rests upon 'Existential-phenomenological tenets and concepts' (1998, p. 14; 1981), and she too cites Heidegger and Merleau-Ponty. Similarly, Jean Watson's (1979) work also claims such a basis.

Several nurse scholars have discussed philosophical concepts and views in order to advance claims concerning the nature of nursing. Sally Gadow, for example, has written on the relationship between the body and the self (1982), and she also is another figure who supports her views by appeal to the work of Merleau-Ponty and also Hegel (1894).

In the early 1980s Ruth Schröck wrote two extremely significant papers (1981a, b) on the relevance of philosophical enquiry to nursing. Notable figures such as Gortner (1990), Meleis (1985), Silva (see Silva and Rothbart, 1984) and Carper (1978) have also applied elements of academic philosophy in order to support nursing-related claims (see also King and Fawcett, 1997). And recently Jan Reed and Ian Ground published probably the first general introduction to the study of the relationship between philosophy and nursing (1997). It is worth commenting that journals such as *Image, Advances in Nursing Science, Nursing Science Quarterly,* and *Journal of Advanced Nursing* also publish papers of a philosophical nature very frequently.

In 1989 the Institute for Philosophical Research in Nursing was established by Professor June Kikuchi and Dr Helen Simmons at the University of Alberta, Canada. The Institute has hosted several conferences on the philosophy of nursing which have led to the publication of important edited texts on the subject (Kikuchi and Simmons, 1992, 1994; Kikuchi et al., 1996).

In the UK, the University of Brighton hosted an international conference in philosophy of nursing during the 1990s, and several such conferences have since taken place at University of Wales, Swansea. More recently, a journal with an explicit remit to publish papers within philosophy of nursing has also appeared (*Nursing Philosophy*), and so has a Web-based discussion page (nurse-philosophy@mailbase.ac.uk).

These brief observations put into context the way the relationship between philosophy and nursing has developed, largely since the 1960s. And a body of work and interests which warrants the title of 'philosophy of nursing' has begun to emerge.

As has become evident, the enterprise of philosophy of nursing *need not* involve the specific proposal of 'philosophies' of nursing in Marriner-Tomey's sense of that term. Rather it has tended to involve much more the kind of analytic and critical activities which are typical of academic philosophy (see, for example, Gadow, 1982; Cash, 1990; Bishop and Scudder, 1991; Kikuchi and Simmons, 1992; Paley, 1996; Reed and Ground, 1997; Edwards, 1998a). It is the burden of the remainder of this book to describe this activity more fully, and also to give a further indication of its nature, and hence of the nature of philosophy of nursing.

Having drawn attention to the way in which philosophy has been embraced, more or less explicitly, into the nursing context, it is worth stressing the following point. Regardless of whether such a development had occurred it would remain the case that nursing rests upon many philosophical assumptions. For example, theories of nursing typically rest upon specific views of what humans are. For Orem, humans are essentially needs-bearers (see Orem, 1987, p. 73), they meet these needs by the performance of self-care activities. Hence, it can be pointed out that humans need food 'in order to remain alive and to function in accord with natural human endowments' (ibid.). Orem also acknowledges that her theory of nursing borrows from philosophical accounts of human agency (ibid.). For Rogers, persons 'and their environments are perceived as irreducible energy fields' (1987, p. 141). According to Roy, the person is viewed as 'an adaptive system with coping mechanisms manifested by the adaptive modes' (1987, p. 38). Moreover, she also states that her 'model' rests upon certain 'philosophical assumptions' (Roy, 1987, p. 37).

Given what has been said so far then it is evident that any 'philosophy of nursing' in the sense proliferated by Marriner-Tomey – that is, as a general view of the ends and means of nursing – will involve the making of philosophical assumptions. In other words, the proposal of a philosophy of nursing rests upon answers to philosophical questions, for example, relating to the nature of persons, knowledge, care, health and so on.

Lastly, in this introductory section, a word about nursing ethics is called for. The main emphasis in the present text is on areas of philosophy other than nursing ethics – although there are two chapters on care. The reason for this is that the relevance of ethics to nursing is now well recognised (see for example, the journal *Nursing Ethics*, established in 1994). However, the relevance of other areas of philosophy to nursing is not quite so well known. And, at least initially, just as nurses needed to be encouraged and trained to recognise the moral dimension of theory and practice, it can be contended that a similar phase of initial encouragement is needed in order for parallel recognition of the importance of philosophical questions relevant to nursing practice.

Philosophical enquiry

But what makes a question philosophical in nature, as opposed to, say, empirical? Put simply, empirical questions are those which, at least in principle, can be answered by the use of sensory evidence. Hence a dispute concerning an empirical matter can in principle be resolved by such evidence. For example, if one person claims there are presently 40 cars in the hospital car park and another says there are 42, this empirical dispute can be resolved by counting the number of cars presently in the car park.

Philosophical disputes cannot be resolved in such a manner. For example consider the question 'What is a person?', no amount of counting will provide an answer to this. If we were to count persons this would simply beg the question of what a person is. Including someone in our survey would simply presuppose our own favoured criterion.

In order to obtain a feel for the distinctive nature of philosophical enquiry, consider the following remark by Russell:

> Philosophy… is something intermediate between theology and science. Like theology it consists of speculation on matters as to which definite knowledge has, so far, been unascertainable; but like science it appeals to human reason rather than to [for example divine] authority… Between theology and science there is a No Man's Land…, this No Man's Land is philosophy (1939, p. 10).

A number of things of importance are to be found in Russell's statement. For example, consider the way in which disputes are resolved within theology and science on the one hand, and philosophy on the other. Russell suggests that the 'court of appeal' or criterion for resolution of disputes about theological matters is simply religious authority. Typically this is drawn from revelations to certain recognised figures, or from religious texts.

In science, the relevant court of appeal for resolving disputes is empirical evidence. For example, a dispute concerning the melting point of a particular metal can be resolved by devising a test situation to test the rival claims and determine which is correct.

Philosophical disputes seem resolvable in neither of these ways. For example, appeals to authority carry no weight in philosophical debate (or ought not to). Berkeley ridiculed philosophers who appealed to the authority of Aristotle with the statement 'Aristotle hath said it' (*Principles of Human Knowledge*, introduction, para. xx). In philosophical debate any appeal to authority can be queried on the grounds that the said authority may be mistaken.

Nor does empirical evidence carry the weight, in philosophy, which it does in the resolution of scientific disputes. For example, suppose in a debate in moral philosophy, regarding how people ought to behave, it is said, 'Well, most people behave in this way'. This invites the rejoinder: 'Well, most people might be mistaken'. It does not follow from the fact that most people behave in way *w*, that it is right to behave in that way. Similarly, it can be pointed out that the fact that most, or all, people believe something to be true is not sufficient for its being true. Most people used to believe the Earth to be stationary, yet we are now told this is mistaken.

The main similarities and differences between philosophy, and theology and science which Russell's statement helps to bring out may be summarised as follows.

In common with science, appeals to authority are not sufficient to resolve philosophical disputes, and the use of reasoning and inference have a high value. But an important difference between philosophical and scientific enquiry centres on the weight carried by appeals to empirical evidence. In science these can have decisive force, but in philosophy appeals to empirical evidence are not decisive.

With reference to theology, in common with this, philosophical enquiry is often concerned with highly general, speculative questions, for example: What are persons? Can we know anything? How should people act if they want to lead a good life? and so on. Also, in common with theology, appeals to empirical evidence have little role in the resolution of disputes. A main point of difference between theology and philosophy centres on the force of appeals to authority. As we have heard, these carry no weight in philosophical debate.

Finally, we might note that the most weighty ground of religious belief is that of faith. Officially at least, this has no proper role in philosophical enquiry; it is constrained, in the main, by reason alone, although empirical considerations might be recruited to support particular views. So Russell's remark gives us something of the flavour of philosophical enquiry.

There is a further characteristic of such enquiry to which we might usefully draw attention. This is that philosophy is typically concerned with questions of a second-order nature. The second-order character of philosophical enquiry is a feature noted by many commentators (for example Bird, 1972, p. 16; Quinton, 1995, p. 666). Quinton gives the example of claims to knowledge. Here first-order enquiry involves 'acquiring knowledge', for example, perhaps as one might suppose scientists or nurse researchers do in summarising the findings of empirical research. But second-order (that is, philosophical) enquiry into such first-order activity may involve, for example, examination of what it is to be said to 'know' something. What criteria of knowledge are being applied when researchers claim to know that (say) 80 per cent of people suffer from anxiety before going to the dentists, or that there are nine planets in the solar system, or that the moon causes tidal flow on the Earth, and so on?

To give another example, an epidemiologist may report the incidence of schizophrenia in a given population. This is a first-order claim. Second-order enquiry into it might usefully focus on what is meant by 'schizophrenia'. It is plain that the first-order enquiry presupposes some agreed definition of this condition. Does that definition withstand critical scrutiny? Such scrutiny constitutes an enquiry at the second-order level.

To give other examples: suppose it is said 'Smith is better now'. What is meant by 'better'? Or 'Smith is healthy'. What is meant by 'healthy'? Or, 'Smith is a good nurse'. What is meant by 'is a good nurse'? These are all second-order questions. Answers to them are presupposed at the first-order level. Answers to first-order questions will be inadequate if the answers to the second-order queries they provoke are inadequate. For example, if asked why it is judged that Smith is a good nurse, we are told that she is a good nurse because she obeys instructions, we might query the understanding the speaker has of what being a good nurse involves.

It is, of course, possible to construct innumerable other examples of this contrast between first- and second-order expressions. But the above examples should give a flavour of the contrast. Something which is presupposed at the first-order level may become the subject of enquiry at the second-order level. This may involve an enquiry into what knowledge is, what a person is, what schizophrenia is, what a good nurse is, what acting wrongly involves and so on.

It is also worth noting that it is characteristic of second-order level enquiry that it focuses on what is meant by key terms in first-order claims ('know', 'nurse', 'health' and so on). Again, this is typical of such enquiry because it is the conditions for the correct application of such terms, the coherence of the terms, or the question of what is referred to by those terms, which are often investigated. Hence the question: 'What is meant by...?' is a key, second-order philosophical question.

A well-known example of study at this level in nursing is Dickoff and James' (1968) paper 'A theory of theories: a position paper'. They examine the conditions which a theory of nursing must satisfy. Hence, they are not producing a theory of nursing (that is, a first-order enterprise), rather they examine from the second-order perspective the very idea of a theory of nursing. A paper by Cash (1990) conducts a similar enquiry into the very idea of a nursing model.

So far then, we have identified something of the nature of philosophical enquiry: it differs importantly from scientific and theological modes of enquiry. And we have noted further that philosophical questions typically have a second-order character. We now proceed to outline four main areas of enquiry within philosophy. In doing so we will signal problems within each area which seem relevant to nursing. The four areas are epistemology, ontology, value-enquiry, and logic.

Epistemology

The province of this is the concept of knowledge. Traditional problems here include the following three. First, the problem of establishing a criterion for knowledge, for example, in order to distinguish knowledge from belief. Second, the problem relating to sources of knowledge, for example, can the senses or reason, or intuition provide knowledge? And third, can we distinguish differing types of knowledge, for example practical and theoretical, moral, aesthetic and others?

To see how problems in epistemology arise in nursing, consider these observations. Given the choice of basing nursing interventions on what is known to be effective as opposed to what is merely believed to be so, it is reasonable to suppose it preferable to ground interventions on what is known. This raises at least two types of question.

What definition of knowledge should be invoked in such a distinction? As we will see in Chapter 2, well-grounded beliefs can be shown to fall short of knowledge. If this is so, how can one distinguish well-grounded beliefs from knowledge? Should claims to know be more properly expressed as beliefs?

Also, what is the relationship between knowledge of 'facts' – propositional knowledge – and the knowledge involved in skilled, practical activities? What are the criteria which determine the possession of such practical knowledge? Are such criteria bound to success in the performance of such acts?

This raises a central and difficult area of enquiry. The question of the effectiveness of a nursing intervention cannot be answered independently of some conception of what the ends of nursing are, of the whole point of nursing. Plausible candidates for this include the relief of suffering, promotion of well-being, fostering autonomy, and perhaps others. Yet 'objective' (that is, independent) knowledge of them appears problematic since the question of whether or not they are met seems inseparable from the patient's own view of the matter, from her own private perspective on her own experiences.

Still within the province of epistemology, are there special sources of knowledge such as 'intuition' which expert nurses access in their practice? This is a view associated with the work of Benner and one we consider below (Chapter 3).

More generally, which methods are best suited to gaining knowledge and understanding of nursing phenomena, positivist, interpretivist, realist or some other? We consider the suitability of these in Chapter 8.

Certain of these questions will be taken up in later chapters, notably chapters 2 and 3 which focus on discussion of the idea of knowledge in the nursing context.

Ontology

The second main area of philosophy mentioned above, is that of ontology. Standard problems within this field include: Does the world exist independently of human thought? Or is its existence inseparable from it? What are persons? Do persons have free will? What is time? What is space? What is an object? and so on. It is characteristic of ontological enquiry to seek to uncover the defining features of the objects of its enquiry, for example persons, space, time and so on.

With reference to nursing, ontological problems which seem relevant include the following. What are persons? Are they mere biological organisms? Or are they 'more than' this? As will be seen in Chapter 4, answers to such questions bear centrally upon questions regarding the nature of nursing.

Also, to give further examples of how ontological enquiry is relevant to nursing, in diagnosing disease are we describing that which really exists, or simply imposing an essentially arbitrary system of categories on to the world? If we think the latter, how should denials of illness be responded to? If we suppose disease to be 'real', an answer seems available. But if disease is not real, only imposed, is the compulsory treatment of disease morally reprehensible, the arbitrary imposition of power on politically weak individuals? These questions indicate the way in which judgements within ontology can inform moral judgements, for example concerning the legitimacy of compulsory treatment.

Relatedly, in trying to establish what 'the meaning' of an illness is for a patient, does this entail that there is such a 'real meaning'? If there is, can it be determined what this is? What view of meaning is presupposed in such claims?

Some nurse commentators seem sympathetic to a view such that the nature of reality is determined by people's conception of it. How are phenomena such as delusions and hallucinations to be accommodated within such a view? The very intelligibility of these categories seems to trade upon a distinction between how things seem and how things really are.

Value-enquiry

The third area of philosophical enquiry is that of value-enquiry, the main components of which are ethics and aesthetics. These are properly described as part of the province of value-enquiry since they concern judgements which are value judgements. Moral judgements appear to express the values of the judger. A judgement that an action *a* is right or good indicates that the person making the judgement values actions of type *a*. Similarly with aesthetic judgements; a judgement that a work of art *a* is better than another work of art *b* seems to imply that *a* is valued more highly than *b*.

With specific reference to nursing, since Carper's important paper 'Fundamental patterns of knowing in nursing' (1978) attempts have been made to try to develop the claim that there is, in a non-trivial sense, an aesthetic element to nursing. Is this a plausible view? On the face of it, the domains of nursing and art seem far apart. This is an issue we return to in Chapter 3 and also in Chapter 9.

With reference to ethics, as noted earlier, this has received very considerable attention within nursing literature in the past thirty years at least. But what precisely is the status of the ethical dimension to nursing practice? Is it part of nursing, by definition, or can there be nursing without such an aspect? Is the ethical dimension intrinsic or foundational, or some other?

More importantly perhaps, what approach to moral problems should nurses adopt? Should their moral reasoning be informed by moral principles or a sense of care, or some fusion of these? Is generalisation possible within ethics as it applies to nursing? Or, once more, given the importance of individual narratives must ethical problems always be viewed anew, so to speak, with no generalisation possible? And which is the ethically appropriate position? One of involvement or detachment, or some other?

Issues relating to moral perception, the place of emotion in ethics, the significance of suffering, and the idea of 'moral phenomenology' have all seemed important (legitimately so) to various nurse philosophers.

Logic

The fourth and final area of philosophy to be mentioned here is that of logic. Crudely, this involves an enquiry into argumentation itself: into the relations of implication which hold between the patterns of claims which comprise arguments. The focus of logic is not on the details of specific arguments or sets of claims, but rather on the form of such arguments.

I will not attempt to expand upon the relevance of logic to nursing. It seems plausible to suppose that reasoning within nursing (and elsewhere!) should respect basic logical principles, notably that relating to the importance of avoiding contradictions in one's reasoning. But the status of this too as a constraint on reasoning has been called into question in recent years by a significant number of nurse writers. Does slavish adherence to the principle simply betray a commitment and 'privileging' of a crude 'binarism' typical of Western, male thought – a commitment which can be challenged from neglected, hidden perspectives, for example those of women and other oppressed groups?

Of course this run through the four main areas of philosophical enquiry has not listed all possible philosophical problems relevant to nursing. My aim has been merely to give an illustration of the nature of the four areas and a brief pointer to areas within each which seem central to nursing. In subsequent chapters we focus on epistemology (Chapters 2 and 3) and on ontology (Chapters 4, 5 and 7). As noted the realm of value-enquiry arises in our discussion of Carper (Chapter 3) and also in Chapter 6 concerning the concept of care.

So far then, following a brief historical introduction, we have attempted to glean something of the flavour of philosophical enquiry. We considered a remark of Russell's which further illuminates the nature of philosophical enquiry. The second-order character of philosophical questions was considered briefly together with some illustrative examples. We then looked at the four main areas of philosophy. It quickly became evident that each of these main areas raises questions of central concern to nursing.

Two useful philosophical tools

Lastly in this section, the pursuance of philosophical enquiry is aided by the use of two philosophical tools which will be appealed to throughout the remainder of the book.

The first of these recruits a distinction between those characteristics of things which define them, and those which are peripheral to them. The second is a distinction between necessary and sufficient conditions.

Some readers may prefer to skip the following on the grounds that knowledge gleaned about tools is best gained from using them. However, it is incumbent upon me to provide a description of the tools here which can be referred back to as necessary. Also, as will be seen, the tools themselves raise a rather thorny problem which I have dealt with in a lengthy note below.

The distinction between necessary and contingent truths

A distinction can be drawn between statements which are *necessarily* true of a thing, and statements which are *contingently* true of that thing. For example, consider the number 2. It is necessarily true of that number that it is an even number (being an even number is a property the number 2 must necessarily possess; anything which is said to be the number 2 must be an even number). This could not be otherwise.

Suppose the number 2 happens to be my lucky number (I always pick it in the lottery, say). It is only *contingently* true of the number 2 that it is my lucky number. My lucky number could have been *any* number, or I might not have had a lucky number at all. So being my lucky number is only contingently true of the number 2. This can be contrasted with the statement '2 is an even number' which, as we saw, is necessarily true of the number 2.

The distinction between necessary and contingent truth helps bring out features of things which are central to them, which define them. If we can identify a statement which is *necessarily* true of a thing – which is true of that thing by definition so to speak – we can be confident that the statement describes something more central to the thing's nature than a statement which is only contingently true of a thing.

The distinction is of particular relevance in philosophical enquiry since in that, one is typically attempting to uncover that which is central to whatever it is one is investigating: that is, to uncover that which is necessarily true of the object of investigation, rather than merely contingently true of it.

The distinction provides us with a tool which we can employ to uncover the nature of nursing, and which we can employ to assess claims concerning the nature of nursing. In such an enquiry we want to uncover that which is fundamental to nursing, that which defines it, is necessarily true of it, as opposed to that which is peripheral, or contingently true of it. For example, statements such as 'nursing involves the performance of caring actions', or 'nursing is a science' seem candidates for necessary truths about nursing. Statements such as 'nurses tend to live in flats' or 'nurses wear headbands' or 'I was once a nurse' seem unlikely candidates for necessary truths about nursing. They don't point to its very nature: they are contingently true, at best, of nursing.

In subsequent chapters we will employ the distinction in pursuit of questions relating to the nature of nursing, the nature of caring, and the nature of persons, among others.

It should be said that the idea of the distinction between necessary and contingent truths has been called into question in recent years (see, for example, Smith, 1997). It has been argued that, very strictly speaking, no statements are necessarily true of a thing, only contingently so. For our purposes we can set this controversy aside. What is central for our purposes is to note that some statements describe aspects of things which are central to them, while others describe only peripheral aspects of things.[1]

Necessary and sufficient conditions

A further distinction which we will make use of during what follows is that between conditions which are necessary for the instantiation of a concept, and conditions which are sufficient for its instantiation. This distinction can be described as follows. Necessary conditions are those which any instance of a concept cannot fail to exemplify. Thus, it is said that the presence of oxygen is a necessary condition for the presence of fire (apparently, combustion cannot occur without oxygen). If this is true, oxygen is a necessary condition of fire. Sufficient conditions are those the presence of which ensure the occurrence of something. Thus if s is a sufficient condition of a, the presence of s guarantees the presence of a: a cannot fail to materialise. Given this, it is clear that oxygen cannot be a sufficient condition for the occurrence of fire, for the presence of oxygen does not bring about the occurrence of fire. Other factors need to be present – for example heat of a particular level, and fuel. Flew puts the distinction as follows:

This is a *necessary condition* for that if, and only if, that cannot be without this. This is a *sufficient condition* for that if, and only if, this is by itself enough to guarantee that (1979, p. 242).

Once again, the distinction will occur throughout what follows, and will be seen to be especially relevant to our discussions of knowledge, care, and the nature of nursing. With these preliminaries complete, we now move on to say more concerning the nature of philosophy of nursing.

Philosophy of nursing

The points made so far in this chapter enable us to draw three fairly robust conclusions concerning the kind of enquiry which constitutes philosophy of nursing.

First, as noted, philosophical questions which nursing throws up are not resolvable solely by empirical means. Thus questions concerning personhood, health, knowledge, care, and illness although central to conceptions of nursing require philosophical thought.

Second, since philosophy is concerned with second-order questions, so too will philosophy of nursing. Thus its concern will focus on those first-order statements, acceptance of which the coherence of nursing rests upon (for example, regarding nursing, knowledge, persons, care, and health).

Lastly, by way of providing a 'nutshell' definition of philosophy of nursing here is one which seems useful: Philosophy of nursing is the examination of philosophical problems as these bear upon, or are raised by, nursing theory and practice. I would suggest that this definition suggests strong parallels with other areas of philosophy such as philosophy of religion, sport, psychology, and science. For these sub-disciplines within philosophy all stem from examination of philosophical problems as these bear upon, or are raised by, religion, sport, psychology and science respectively.

What I would like to do now is to try to articulate a fairly rough, but hopefully useful, distinction between three strands of enquiry in philosophy of nursing.

A philosophical presuppositions strand

This involves a focus on the basic assumptions of nursing discourse. So, for example, Carper and Benner each make certain assumptions regarding the nature of knowledge in their work. This strand of work within philosophy of nursing involves the identification and assessment of such presuppositions. Thus having identified that Carper, say, presupposes a certain conception of knowledge, it can be asked whether this conception is in fact a credible one.

Clearly if it is not, then the claims based upon the relevant conception seem vulnerable to serious criticism. As we will see below (Chapter 3), Carper's work does seem to involve presuppositions regarding knowledge, and also aesthetics, which invite criticism.

So the relevant task here is a more self-consciously nursing task. It involves the examination of important texts in nursing discourse, seeking to expose their philosophical presuppositions, and assessing their legitimacy. As we heard above, such texts will inevitably involve the presumption of answers to some philosophical questions (for example, regarding the nature and scope of knowledge).

Further examples of such presuppositions include claims regarding the nature and ends of nursing. Any claim regarding the nature of nursing presupposes an answer to the second-order, philosophical question: 'What is nursing?' Any answer to this will inevitably involve some view of the means and ends of nursing. A focus on likely candidates for the ends of nursing, say, will rapidly bring us to consideration of concepts such as suffering, well-being, disease, health, illness, autonomy and others. Which view of these concepts is presupposed in the view of nursing being subjected to philosophical scrutiny? So, setting aside a focus on means, it is evident that any general view of nursing will lend itself to scrutiny from within this strand of philosophy of nursing.

In addition to the kinds of enquiries just identified, such work would also usefully focus on attempts to plot the relations between theories, models, philosophies, paradigms and metaparadigms of nursing. For example, with regard to the sense of the term 'philosophy' in nursing, as noted earlier, there is a tendency to employ this as a synonym of theory. This causes some confusion for then philosophy of nursing is considered to amount to providing theories of nursing. But, this is not so. Or, at least, there is another perfectly proper use of the term 'philosophy' which does not involve the proposal of nursing theories. Rather, philosophy of nursing is at a level prior to the development of nursing theories. For, as suggested above, any nursing theory will involve philosophical commitments. For example, regarding personhood, care, health, illness, and knowledge.

A philosophical problems strand

Two phases of this can be discerned. First, having identified philosophical presuppositions in the manner described in the first strand, rather than deliberate completely anew in relation to these, use can be made of existing philosophical literature on the relevant topic (if there is any). Thus, to return to the example of Carper's work, once her presuppositions regarding the nature of knowledge have been identified, existing philosophical work on that topic can be turned to in order to shed light on Carper's views. Such philosophical work may offer ways of refining Carper's claims so they are less vulnerable to criticism.

To take another example, suppose it is agreed that alleviating suffering should figure among the ends of nursing. Suppose further, by application of the philosophical presuppositions strand, it emerges that a theorist holds a specific conception of suffering. The consideration of existing philosophical work on that topic may illuminate further ways of understanding suffering. If there is a conflict between the various positions, which is the more plausible position?

In short, this first phase of enquiry within our 'philosophical problems' strand is intended to avoid the necessity for those who have pursued the first strand to 'reinvent the wheel'. If useful philosophical work is already extant on a specific topic, why not make use of it? This, of course, is not to say that the philosophical work should be presumed correct or more authoritative than the view of the relevant nurse writer.

The second phase of enquiry in our philosophical problems strand is prompted by the observation that it requires a considerable amount of work simply to recognise philosophical issues in nursing. One way to aid this process of recognition is to consider how traditional philosophical problems – for example relating to knowledge, or relations between mind and body, and so on – bear upon nursing. Part of the reason why this seems to me a difficult task is that if one wants to discover what the standard problems of philosophy are, one can turn to any number of books on that subject. But there are few books concerning the problems of philosophy of nursing (except Reed and Ground, 1997; Edwards, 1998a).

The fourfold division of philosophy described above should help to illustrate the nature of this specific strand of enquiry within philosophy of nursing. It involves discussion of problems within the various areas of philosophy as these bear upon nursing. Thus activity within this strand of philosophy of nursing may focus on problems relating to knowledge, ontology, values and logic. Those pursuing philosophy of nursing might usefully draw upon work done previously in such areas within philosophy in their attempts to resolve the problems they generate within nursing. As mentioned, discussion within this strand figures significantly in the present volume when we focus on knowledge, care, persons and so on.

A 'scholarship' strand

In addition to the two strands of philosophy of nursing just mentioned, a third can be added. This can described as a 'scholarship' strand. This involves the assessment of claims made by nurse-theorists for a philosophical basis for their respective views.

As noted above, it has become common in nursing literature to identify the works of particular philosophers or philosophical movements as providing a philosophical basis for a particular theory of nursing. Frequently, references are made to Husserl, Heidegger, Merleau-Ponty, and numerous other philosophers, or to the phenomenological or 'existential-phenomenological' traditions in philosophy.

It seems to me to be an important component of philosophy of nursing to assess the legitimacy of such claims. This would clearly require examination of the philosophical work of the relevant philosopher. Unless this is done, it is not possible to evaluate the claim that a philosophical position provides a foundation for a nursing theory. (Which is not to say that any nursing theory *need* align itself with any particular philosopher or philosophical movement. What matters more is whether the philosophical presuppositions are coherent and plausible.)

Also, an evaluation of the congruence between the nursing theory and the philosophical views of the named philosopher or philosophical movement is required. For example, suppose in developing a nursing theory a key role was accorded to the autonomy of patients and clients. And suppose the philosophical basis for the theory is the work of a determinist philosopher who denies the existence of free will. Here there is a clear lack of congruence – an inconsistency – between the nursing theory and the philosophical basis claimed for it.

I am not suggesting that any nurse theorist has committed such an error. This is merely an exemplification of the kind of enquiry or scholarship which comprises this strand of philosophy of nursing.

To take an actual example of such work, in his paper 'Husserl, phenomenology and nursing' (1997), John Paley undertakes the kind of task to which I am referring. He points out that many nurse researchers claim their research is grounded in 'Husserlian phenomenology'. However, Paley argues, many such researchers radically misconceive key elements of Husserl's philosophical apparatus, such as the phenomenological reduction.

In Husserl's phenomenological reduction he seeks to place the existence of external objects in abeyance – to refrain from assuming that there are such objects (1931, p. 98). Given this, it seems that attempts to deploy the phenomenological reduction in research into the experiences of other people (for example their experiences of the interventions of nurses) is contradictory. For, any such empirical enquiry presupposes the existence of other people and it is precisely any such presupposition which Husserl wants to rule out in the phenomenological reduction.

The discussion of ontological care below (Chapter 7) can also be regarded as an example of this strand of philosophy of nursing. As will be seen, Benner and Wrubel's appeal to Heidegger's use of 'care' as a central concept in their approach to nursing masks a key distinction between ontological and intentional care.

So, the suggestion here is that a rough but hopefully useful threefold division can be articulated which identifies various strands within philosophy of nursing. The division is rough in the sense that there are clear overlaps between the strands. Thus for example, work in the 'philosophical problems' strand may overlap with that in the 'presuppositions' strand. As seen, the concept of a person is central to most nursing theories and conceptions of nursing. So proper examination of the role of such conceptions will inevitably lead one into the pursuance of enquiry under the 'philosophical problems' strand. This 'slippage' is evident in our discussion of persons in Chapters 4 and 5 below.

Before concluding this chapter, I would like to make a few remarks concerning the 'location' of philosophy of nursing within philosophical enquiry in general.

The conceptual location of philosophy of nursing

What is the place of philosophy of nursing within the discipline of philosophy? Philosophy of nursing seems best described, along with philosophy of medicine, as a branch of philosophy of health care. And, philosophy of health care can be described as a branch of applied philosophy.

The reason why philosophy of nursing seems best categorised as a branch of applied philosophy is that nursing is clearly a practical discipline. And, for those involved in practical disciplines it is judged, typically, that any thinking at the theoretical level is only legitimate in so far as it has ramifications for practice. Hence, I suspect that most nurses who become interested in philosophy of nursing do so in the hope that there will be some eventual benefit for nursing practice.

But of course, some people may be interested in the problems of philosophy of nursing simply for their own sakes, regardless of their ramifications for practice. So, for example, a person might be interested in the phenomenon of 'care in nursing' from a philosophical perspective without being concerned about any implications for practice which may arise from various analyses of care. It seems to me that such a person would still be engaged in philosophy of nursing, regardless of whether the person was concerned with implications for practice.

The distinction between applied and non-applied (pure (?)) philosophy is not a simple one and I don't want to spend too much time discussing it here (see Upton, 1998). But the claim advanced here that philosophy of nursing is a branch of applied philosophy seems to be in agreement with the description of applied philosophy given in the *Journal of Applied Philosophy*. The official remit of that journal is to 'provide a focus for philosophical research which has a direct bearing on areas of practical concern' (quoted from the aims of the journal printed on the inside cover of each issue, for example Vol. 10(2), 1993). It seems, then, that much philosophy of nursing fits this description of applied philosophy. For example, Benner's work on expertise (1984), and Gadow's work on the importance of the body (1982) clearly have a direct bearing on an area of practical concern – namely, nursing practice.

On a related matter, it is pertinent to wonder what the direction of influence is between philosophy and nursing? As with others raised in this introductory chapter, this is a large question to which a short answer will be inadequate. But it can be argued that philosophy too has something to gain from considering the kinds of problems which arise in the nursing context. It seems reasonable to claim that adequate understanding of the phenomena of illness, disease and suffering, for example, is more likely if grounded in appreciation of the actual experiences of these aspects of health care work. Similar claims can be made for the appreciation of the significance of the body in the understanding of what it is to be a person. In the moral sphere, the moral phenomenology of nursing seems an important source for the development of understanding of moral philosophy. As a practice discipline, nursing seems an important source of reflection on the nature of practical knowledge. And lastly, the problem of understanding human beings is also, as seen, crucial to nursing. Reflection on this general problem within philosophy of science might usefully be fostered by focusing on the nursing domain.

However, the main purpose of this book is to try to present an introduction to philosophy of nursing. So its main emphasis is on showing how philosophy is relevant to nursing, rather than to mount the case for the claim that nursing is relevant to philosophy.

Having now provided some groundwork on the nature of philosophy, and philosophy of nursing, we turn in the next chapter to a concept fundamental to nursing, that of knowledge.

SUGGESTIONS FOR FURTHER READING

General introductions to philosophy

It is always difficult to give recommendations of this kind since people differ widely on what they find accessible and interesting. However, a very brief but accessible and useful general introduction to philosophy is provided by Thomas Nagel (1987) *What Does it All Mean? A Very Short Introduction to Philosophy*, Oxford: Oxford University Press. This is very much a 'philosophical problems oriented' approach rather than a 'who said what' approach.

At a different level altogether, a much more advanced book is one edited by A.C. Grayling (1995) *Philosophy, A Guide Through the Subject*, Oxford: Oxford University Press. This contains articles on some of the main areas of philosophy (epistemology, ethics, metaphysics, logic, philosophy of mind, philosophy of science, and so on) all written by leading contributors to these respective areas. It is also very reasonably priced – although, it should stressed again, the level of discussion is such that not everyone will find this an easy read.

Between these two books, so to speak, is *Philosophy Made Simple* by R.H. Popkin and A. Stroll (1993) (3rd edn), London: Butterworth-Heinemann. This is intended as an introduction to the subject, and has accessible discussions both of philosophical problems (of ethics, knowledge, mind and so on) and the works of the major philosophers (Plato, Aristotle, Descartes, Hume, Kant and so on).

Texts on philosophy of nursing

The edited collections by June Kikuchi and Helen Simmons (1992, 1994), and with Donna Romyn (1996) – each contain accessible papers specifically within the field of philosophy of nursing. These provide a useful 'way in' to philosophy of nursing. Reed and Ground's book (1997) provides a useful, systematic introduction to philosophy of nursing. Bishop and Scudder's (1991) book is extremely clear and well-written, and provides a philosophical case for conceiving of nursing as a practice.

In addition to these, a new book has appeared by J.M. Brencick and G.A. Webster (2000) *Philosophy of Nursing, A New Vision for Health Care*, New York: State University of New York Press. This focuses on the problem of the relationship between the general and the particular in nursing, and contains an interesting focus on the work of Professor Jean Watson.

Lastly, my own edited collection *Philosophical Issues in Nursing* (1998a) also provides a useful indication of the wide range of issues which fall within the topic of philosophy of nursing, and of how they may be dealt with.

2 Nursing knowledge (i): propositional and practical

This chapter and the next centre on the topic of nursing knowledge. The focus of this chapter lies on propositional and practical knowledge. A specific approach to propositional knowledge is endorsed, following Quine (1951), according to which no claim is immune from revision. Given the definition of knowledge endorsed it follows that knowledge of empirical matters, very strictly speaking, is not attainable. However, as shown below, this can be accepted without lapsing into a position in which all knowledge claims are held to be of equal legitimacy. With reference to practical knowledge, the claim for a distinction between this and propositional knowledge is supported, recruiting arguments made by Ryle (1949).

Our discussion within this chapter is a consequence of engaging in the 'philosophical presuppositions' strand of philosophy of nursing identified in Chapter 1. Carper and Benner were identified as nurse scholars who presuppose an understanding of the concept of knowledge, which, as we will see in this chapter is deeply problematic. We postpone discussion of their specific claims until Chapter 3, and now move on here to consider defining propositional knowledge.

Defining propositional knowledge

The idea of nursing knowledge is one which has received a tremendous amount of discussion within nursing scholarship (Carper, 1978; Benner, 1984; Robinson and Vaughan, 1992; Kikuchi et al., 1996). There seem at least four related reasons for this.

The first is that, as noted earlier, placing nursing practice on a basis of what is known seems preferable to basing nursing practice on what is merely believed or supposed. If pre-operative counselling is known to aid post-operative recovery then a nurse might justifiably devote her time to such counselling. But if it is merely believed or supposed that pre-operative counselling aids post-operative recovery, then the justification for giving such counselling is weaker: perhaps the nurse's time could be better occupied with interventions that are known to help patients. Relatedly, suppose it is known that a drug is thera-peutically effective in relation to a specific illness *x*. Suppose further that the drug has some moderately unpleasant side-effects, in spite of its very considerable therapeutic efficacy. Given that the efficacy of the drug is known it is reasonable to judge that a patient suffering from x will be prepared to put up with the side-effects of the drug, in the knowledge that it will cure her of x. But if the therapeutic efficacy of the drug is merely believed or supposed, then the patient may judge the justification for taking it and putting up with its unpleasant side-effects to be much weaker.

So given a choice between basing nursing interventions upon knowledge or belief, it is reasonable to assert that nurses and patients would prefer such interventions to be based upon the former rather than the latter.

A second reason for the interest in nursing knowledge is the view that the articulation of a body of nursing knowledge will contribute very significantly to the articulation of the unique identity of nursing (Parse, 1995, p. 51). Such a body of knowledge might serve to individuate nursing in the way in which, say, astronomy is distinguishable from biology due to the body of knowledge within it.

Third, a further motivation for the focus upon nursing knowledge comes from the educational perspective. If a body of nursing knowledge can be described, then it is this which novices to nursing will be expected to learn during their nurse education.

Finally, a fourth reason for discussing the concept of knowledge stems from a scan of definitions of knowledge which occur within nursing literature (recall our 'scholarship strand' of philosophy of nursing mentioned in Chapter 1). A very influential definition produced by Chinn and Kramer runs thus:

> We use the term 'knowing' to refer to the individual human processes of experiencing the world and comprehending the self and the world in ways that can be brought to some level of conscious awareness... [And we] use the term 'knowledge' to refer to knowing that can be shared or communicated with others (1991, p. 5; cited with approval in McKenna, 1997, p. 24; and in Marriner-Tomey, 1994, p. 3).

Suppose we were to look at this definition as critically as possible. What is wrong with it? Note that the definition of knowledge follows the definition of 'knowing', where for Chinn and Kramer, this includes our experiences of perceiving the world around us. Let us set aside the references to comprehending the self and focus on the claim that perception equals knowing; this clearly seems to be implied by the definition given.

Any such view seems plainly wrong as a moment's reflection shows. When I look at railway lines they appear to converge in the distance, as far as it looks to me when I perceive them. But of course they do not. Similarly, a straight stick appears bent when placed in water, but in fact is not. People see mirages in conditions of extreme heat, and so on. In short, perceiving is not a sufficient condition for knowing.

Given that Chinn and Kramer's definition of knowledge rests upon their definition of knowing, the prospects for them providing an adequate definition of knowledge do not look promising. But let us consider the definition of knowledge they offer. As we heard, for them, knowing amounts to perceiving. So they must hold that knowledge is perception 'that can be shared or communicated with others' (ibid.). Read charitably, this must mean roughly the following: reports of perceptions which are communicable convey knowledge.

This seems plainly wrong. Recall the 'stick in water' example given above, if I say 'That stick is bent' to someone nearby I have communicated to them my 'knowing', and so 'that stick is bent' seems to satisfy Chinn and Kramer's definition of knowledge. Yet given the difference between how things appear and how things really are – recall the railway lines example – my statement 'That stick is bent' is surely a mistake, it is not knowledge: I have a mistaken belief. Other definitions of knowledge which occur within nursing literature could similarly be shown to be vulnerable to criticism, but I will not do this here. Instead I propose to begin the chapter with a philosophical discussion of the concept of knowledge. This will then be applied to two seminal discussions of knowledge within the nursing canon by Carper (1978) and Benner (1984).

Both these writers advance claims regarding the nature of knowledge. For Benner such claims help to articulate phenomena of central importance to nursing (for example practical knowledge), and to elucidate the idea of nursing expertise. Carper, officially at least, seeks to enquire into what it means to know something. And she posits the idea of a 'pattern of knowing'. The point of this is to help to articulate the nature of nursing and the kinds of knowledge which are important within it.

Having said this, it is worth pointing out in advance of our discussion of their work that neither Carper nor Benner spends time defining what they mean by 'knowledge'. Benner distinguishes practical and theoretical knowledge, but she does not offer a definition of knowledge, in contrast to belief for example. The same is true of Carper, which seems a major omission in a paper which aims to devote 'critical attention to the question of what it means to know...' (1978, p. 13).

As will be shown later, then, the discussions of Carper and Benner beg at least the fundamental question of what is meant by 'knowledge'. Carper's paper leaves us with questions concerning what knowledge is, with the view that there are kinds of knowledge, that the idea of a 'pattern of knowing' is a coherent one; and lastly, that a claim can be known at one time, and yet later turn out to be false (1978, p. 22). Benner's work requires us to consider the question of the difference, if any, between practical and theoretical knowledge, and the nature of intuition. With this range of issues in mind we turn now to look more closely at the very idea or concept of knowledge.

Why prefer what is known to what is believed?

It was suggested above that it is knowledge rather than belief which provides a firmer justification for our choices, whether these concern performing one kind of nursing intervention as opposed to another, or a decision to take one kind of medication rather than another. The reason for preferring to base acts upon what is known as opposed to what is believed derives from a criterion by which belief can be distinguished from knowledge. This is that while there is a necessary relationship between knowledge and truth there is only a contingent relationship between belief and truth. In other words, it is a necessary truth that if a person knows something, then what they know must be true. But if a person merely believes something it is not necessarily true that what they believe is true. Thus there is a necessary relationship between knowledge and truth but only a contingent one between belief and truth.

In explanation of this, consider the following two statements:

(a) Smith knows that the nursing lecture begins at 10.00am on 26 February 1999.
(b) Smith believes that the nursing lecture begins at 10.00am on 26 February 1999.

For (a) to be true (that is, for it to be the case that Smith knows the time of the lecture), it has to be the case that the lecture begins at 10.00am. In fact, for any proposition p which is known by someone, it is a necessary condition of their knowing that proposition p is true. (Here we follow the convention of using 'p' to stand for the proposition known or believed.) So the relationship between Smith and what is known is such that Smith only knows something if what he knows is in fact true.

Contrast this with (b). In relation to belief there is no such relationship between what is believed and Smith's believing it. It can be true that Smith believes the lecture begins at 10.00am whether or not it does actually begin then. In fact, it can be true that Smith believes anything, however bizarre, without it being the case that what he believes is true. Smith might believe pigs give birth to human babies, and although it may be true that Smith believes this, it does not follow that pigs do in fact give birth to human babies. But for it to be true that Smith knows that pigs give birth to human babies, it would have to be the case that they did.

Hopefully, then, the claim that knowledge is necessarily related to truth while belief is not is now understood. This helps account for a preference for knowledge over belief. For if we do genuinely know something, then what we know must be true. And for obvious reasons we would rather ground our decisions on what really is true rather than on what simply is believed to be true.

An important consequence

This view of the relationship between knowledge and truth has a rather significant consequence, one which is of particular significance to the nursing context. Kikuchi and Simmons (1996, p. 12) point with disapproval to the emergence within nursing of a specific view of the relationship between knowledge and truth in which knowledge and belief are conflated. In such a view, it is held that if a person believes something is the case, then what they believe is true. An important flaw in such views – in which belief is taken to be sufficient for knowledge – is worth setting out explicitly here.

Consider the two statements (c) and (d) below:

(c) Smith knows that the nursing lecture begins at 10.00am on 26 February 1999.
(d) Jones knows that the nursing lecture begins at 10.30am on 26 February 1999.

Assume Smith and Jones are thinking of the same lecture. Given the necessary relationship between knowledge and truth it follows that Smith and Jones cannot *both* know the time of the lecture. One of them (at least) must be mistaken. Either the lecture starts at 10.00am or 10.30am or some other time. What cannot be true is that the lecture both starts at 10.00am and also that it starts at 10.30am. For the truth of one of these logically excludes the possibility that the other is true. The reason why this truism is spelt out so pedantically here is as follows.

The trend in nursing scholarship to which Kikuchi and Simmons refer is one according to which believing that *p* is true, is sufficient for knowing that *p* is true. This leads to a position in which if A believes/knows the lecture begins at 10.00am then it is claimed to be 'true for A' that the lecture begins at 10.00am. Hence, if B believes/knows the lecture begins at 10.30am it is similarly claimed to be 'true for B' that the lecture begins at 10.30am.

It does not take long to see that such views are highly problematic, even untenable. For example how would communication be possible? One could never suppose any agreed standards or spatio-temporal coordinates. Suppose A and B decide to meet up for coffee. A says to B 'I'll meet you at 6.00pm in the hospital café'. B is there promptly at 6.00pm. A does not show up. B sees A the next day and asks why he didn't make their meeting. A responds: 'It may be true for you that I failed to show up, but it is true for me that I did and that you did not in fact turn up for our planned meeting'.

Such a response is legitimate on the view which conflates knowledge and belief. It is possible to construct much more serious examples of the application of such a view of knowledge to the nursing context. For example it may be 'true for' nurse A that he has fed a patient, but 'true for' the patient that he has not been fed. So the general proposal is being made here that the position in which believing is sufficient for knowing is not in fact a very plausible one, and that its implementation in practice would have disastrous consequences.[1]

A criterion for knowledge

So far, then, we have tried to show that knowledge and belief differ crucially in their relations to truth, and thus to show that belief is not sufficient for knowledge. The reason is of course A's believing that *p* is not sufficient for the truth of *p*, while if we know that A knows that *p*, then we know *p* must be true. (Knowledge entails the truth of what is known; belief does not entail the truth of what is believed.)

Consider now a commonly appealed to 'tripartite' criterion of knowledge put forward to aid the distinction proposed between knowledge and belief. On this criterion knowledge is defined as justified true belief (see, for example, Plato's *Theaetetus* 210c–202d; Moser, 1992).

The criterion states three necessary conditions which any belief must satisfy in order to qualify as knowledge. (a) The first is a 'belief condition'. According to this for it to be true that A knows that *p*, then A must believe that *p*. (b) The second is a 'truth condition' such that for it to be true that A knows that *p*, then *p* must be true. (c) The third condition is the justification condition such that there must be some evidence relating the belief to what is known.

All three conditions are necessary conditions, so on this account A might have a true belief without this amounting to knowledge. What would be lacking would be the justification for holding the belief. Hence suppose A comes to believe his house is burning down, even though A is miles from his home and in receipt of no empirical information which might lead him to such a belief. Suppose further that, as things turn out, A's belief is in fact a true belief (that is, his house is actually burning down). On the tripartite conception of knowledge, A's belief falls short of knowledge. This, I suspect, conforms with our intuitions about what it is to know. If, when pressed, A is unable to point to any justification for his belief, then standardly we would refrain from allowing that A's belief amounts to knowledge.

What this view of knowledge brings out is the relationship between belief and what is believed. For beliefs to count as knowledge, some requirement of evidence is necessary, and this evidence must be appropriately related to what is known. In the case of A's belief that his house is burning down, such evidence might take the form of smoke rising from the area where his house is, or probably something more specific even than this.

Although this account of knowledge seems promising, it has been shown to be open to serious objection. Gettier (1963) sketches examples which call it into question. One of these runs as follows.

Suppose A works in an office in which there is a clock on the wall which is an accurate timekeeper. Overnight, unbeknownst to A, the clock stops at 10.30pm. Coincidentally, at 10.30am the next morning A looks at the clock. Given its general reliability A judges it to be 10.30am. He now has a justified true belief. The belief is true because it is 10.30. The belief is justified since the clock in normally reliable; and, trivially, the belief condition also seems met.

Sceptical worries

Thus Gettier presents a serious challenge to the tripartite model of knowledge with the example just given. Other philosophers have advanced similar challenges to the possibility of our ever obtaining knowledge. In one version of this sceptical challenge, described by Descartes, since at any one time one cannot be sure that one is not dreaming, then it is not possible to obtain the degree of certainty which one would normally require to accompany knowledge. One might believe one is presently sat in front of the computer writing but hasn't one dreamt one was engaged in that activity? How can one be sure that now is not one of those dreams? (See 'First meditation' in Descartes, 1954.)

With reference to the domain of science, Newton-Smith points to a 'pessimistic induction' such that 'any theory will be discovered to be false within, say, 200 years of being propounded' (1981, p. 14). Seemingly unassailable beliefs such as the belief that the Earth is stationary have been overturned and rejected as false. Thus Ptolemy's cosmology was replaced by that of Copernicus, Newton's theories were replaced by Einstein's, and so on. More recently, the view that the cause of sudden infant death syndrome (SIDS) lay within the affected infants was called into question, as was the hypothesis that SIDS has a genetic cause. Now it is held that the cause of SIDS lies beyond the individual infant, and a genetic cause unlikely. This characteristic pattern of theory acceptance and later rejection lends support to the pessimistic induction of which Newton-Smith speaks.

A Quinean response

In the light of this, it might seem that one cannot possess any knowledge at all, certainly with respect to empirical phenomena. However, one response outlined by Quine (1951; Quine and Ullian, 1978; and, within nursing, Booth et al., 1997), is to grant the force of the sceptic's challenge but to deny it follows from this that all beliefs are on an equal footing, so to speak.

For example, it *may* be true that as I am sitting here typing I cannot be absolutely certain that I am not dreaming. But it seems more plausible that I am actually here typing than that I am dreaming. My confidence that I am not dreaming derives from considerations such as the regularity of my present experiences, their taking place in a logical sequence, the absence of deviations from experiences which I take as typical of waking experience, and so on.

Similarly, it is *possible* that the patient one saw two minutes ago has been replaced in bed by an alien which looks exactly like the patient. But is this *likely?* Unless one has particular grounds for suspicion the 'replacement' possibility will not be given serious consideration.

Applied to the scientific domain, Quine's approach recognises that no theories are ever likely to be true, hence he claims 'no statement is immune to revision' (1951, p. 43). So he acknowledges the force of the pessimistic induction. But it remains possible to employ criteria to judge beliefs more or less plausible. As in the response given to the 'dreaming argument', criteria such as regularity and coherence can be recruited in favour of the view that I am not now dreaming. These criteria do not give absolute cast-iron guarantees, only criteria of plausibility. This might be expressed as follows: 'The belief that I am not dreaming has greater epistemic warrant than the belief that I am. So I am more justified in concluding that I am not dreaming than that I am.'

In an attempt to set out such criteria, Quine and Ullian posit desirable traits of beliefs or hypotheses – 'virtues' (1978, p. 66) as they describe them. These run as follows: 'conservatism', 'modesty', 'simplicity', 'generality', and 'refutability' (1978, pp. 66–79). Their suggestion is that these 'virtues' count in favour of the plausibility of a belief or hypothesis.

In summary of these, conservatism requires that we do not readily accept beliefs the acceptance of which would require jettisoning hitherto successful beliefs. Consider this in relation to the alien example. The belief that the patient has been replaced by an identical-looking alien requires the over-turning of the plausible belief that the patient one left momentarily and then returned to, although with the same physical appearance as the patient, is not in fact him. Of course it is *possible* (just about) that the patient has been replaced, but with no evidence to the contrary, one sticks with beliefs which have been successful so far and does not overturn them in favour of untried beliefs (such as the alien example).

With reference to the *limits* of conservatism, consider this example from nursing research. The example helps to show that this 'virtue' need not entail slavish adherence to currently accepted views. It has apparently been shown that the practice of lengthy pre-operative fasting of patients has more harmful consequences than good ones (Booth et al., 1997, p. 809). Adhering to the virtue of conservatism requires that we hold on to the previous belief about pre-operative fasting until there is good evidence in favour of the newer belief. So older, well-established beliefs are presumed plausible, roughly on the grounds that they would have been overturned if they had nothing to count for them, and the burden of proof lies with newer, rival beliefs.

Research into pre-operative fasting shows lengthy fasting to be unnecessary and harmful. Hence, practice can be modified in the light of such research.

Related to conservatism, Quine and Ullian identify *modesty* as a virtue. The more modest belief is that which is the least adventurous, as they put it 'the lazy world is the likely world' (1978, p. 68). In the alien example, the belief that the patient remains the same is clearly the more modest belief. Hence this virtue would also counsel us to dispense with the alien belief.

In relation to the pre-operative fasting example, the new belief is not modest in one way in that it causes us to revise an existing belief. However, acceptance of the new belief does not require extensive revision of a very wide range of existing beliefs (contrast this with the alien example). So although modesty still inclines us to favour currently accepted beliefs, we can see that a modest challenge can be mounted to these, for example of the kind presented by the research on pre-operative fasting.

Simplicity is the third virtue posited (1978, p. 69; also Watson, 1968; Newton-Smith, 1981). In our alien example, the belief that the patient's identity remains the same is clearly the simpler one. And this preference for simpler over complex explanations can be discerned throughout the history of science (for example Watson, 1968).

Assessment of the simplicity of the two rival beliefs about pre-operative fasting would appear to depend upon their relations to other relevant beliefs. For example, relating to time required for digestion of food and liquid. If the typical period of this is four hours, then the simpler belief seems that which recommends a fasting period of not much more than this. The further away from this, for example eight hours, then the less simple the belief.

The fourth virtue is generality. Applied to hypotheses, Quine and Ullian state: 'The wider the range of application of a hypothesis, the more general it is' (p. 73). Thus if one considers the statement 'The sum of the internal angles of a triangle always total 180 degrees', this is a statement with staggering generality. It applies to every triangle. Or consider the hypothesis to the effect that a treatment cures all cases of a specific illness, against a hypothesis that it will cure only one such case. The point is that the more general hypothesis, from a scientific perspective, is considered the more desirable, for obvious reasons.

Take the example of pre-operative fasting again. Suppose there are two theories, one which applies only to male adults, and excludes females, the other which applies to all adults. The second theory is the more general, and on this account the preferred theory, if it does in fact apply to all adults, male or female. A still more general theory would apply to all mammals.

This virtue does not easily apply to our alien example. But it is worth noting that it seems more plausible to cling to the more general belief that 'patients are not replaced by aliens' than the belief that 'this patient has been replaced by an alien'.

The final virtue which Quine and Ullian posit is 'refutability' (1978, p. 79). With reference to the empirical domain, and hence to practice disciplines such as nursing, this seems an important requirement of beliefs. Suppose it is claimed, as before, that pre-operative fasting has hitherto deprived patients of food for a needlessly long period of time. Before we embark upon a programme of reducing the period of pre-operative fasting, it seems appropriate to try to test the claim. This of course requires that the claim is in fact testable; which in turn requires that it can either be confirmed or shown to be false.

An example of a non-refutable belief helps to see why refutability is thought by Quine and Ullian to be a virtue of beliefs (see also Popper, 1963). Consider: 'Pre-operative fasting periods of four hours either do or do not increase the risk of inhalation of gastric contents during anaesthesia'. This is plainly not a refutable claim. It is true whether or not pre-operative fasting periods of four hours increase the risk of inhalation of gastric contents. Hence, from a practice point of view the claim is uninformative. Put another way, the claim is empirically empty since it is compatible with all possible outcomes, and rules no outcomes out.

With regard to our alien example, the belief that the patient has been replaced by an alien at least satisfies this virtue: the belief is refutable. By conducting relevant investigations we can determine whether the patient is a human or an alien.

So this approach to knowledge, in effect, concedes that knowledge may not be possible to obtain but denies that all beliefs are, therefore, on an equal footing. Some beliefs can be supported by evidence which gives us grounds to take them as more plausible than other beliefs for which there is no evidence, or only unconvincing evidence. Beliefs which satisfy the virtues identified by Quine and Ullian have more going for them than beliefs which do not.

It should be said that this approach to knowledge is not uncontroversial. Some philosophers think the sceptic's challenges can be resisted, and there are difficulties internal to the Quinean approach (for example regarding the virtue of conservatism, does not this militate against acceptance of new beliefs?). However, it seems to me to be quite a helpful approach to episte-mological issues in the nursing context (with limitations to be discussed below). The reason is this. Within the approach, beliefs are expected to be supported by the provision of reasons. Of course the provision of evidence in support of a claim would count as a reason in favour of adopting it.

The expectation that knowledge claims be justified by reasons seems crucial in the nursing context, for example in relation to new treatments or new types of nursing interventions. It seems a proper requirement on practice that it can be supported by reason, such as may be provided by empirical evidence. It also seems reasonable that any proposed changes in practice should have to be justi-fied in some way, again, for example by the provision of evidence.

So within this Quinean approach, beliefs are expected to be supportable by the provision of reasons. And if one approach to nursing practice has evidence in support of it and another has not, then there are prima facie grounds for adopting the first approach in preference to the other. In short, adoption of the first approach is then justified by appeal to reasons.

Further, within this Quinean approach, no beliefs are considered 'sacred' or immune from revision as Quine puts it. Thus no practices can be expected to be exempt from scrutiny on the grounds that they have always been in place (see Rodgers on dogma in nursing practice, 1991). Again, this seems a welcome approach to health care work.

So the broadly Quinean approach to knowledge which is being put forward here is one which, first of all, recognises that our ways of doing nursing practice are essentially revisable. If a better approach is found then that should be adopted, where 'better' here means an approach which more appropriately meets the ends of nursing.

And lastly, it should be stressed that the Quinean approach to knowledge places important emphasis upon the role of evidence in support of beliefs: appeals to tradition, authority and dogma are not sufficient to warrant acceptance of beliefs. The provision of evidence, in contrast, can provide support. (Although as we will see later, the idea of evidence requires considerable qualification in the nursing context.)

In summary: the two main points which are to be taken from this discussion are these. First, that there is a crucial distinction to be recognised between knowledge and belief. And second, the point that although all we seem left with are beliefs, these can be evaluated in terms of their varying degrees of plausibility (this to be determined by reference to evidential considerations and the criteria advanced by Quine and Ullian and discussed above).

Our discussion so far has said nothing on the topic of practical knowing. And as noted earlier, this too has been the centre of considerable attention within nursing scholarship. Hence we turn now to discuss the idea of practical knowledge, or 'knowing how' as it is sometimes termed.

Practical knowledge

Our discussion in the last section focused exclusively on propositional knowledge; that is, on what it is to know that a specific proposition is true. But it is common to point out that nursing, as a practical discipline, requires practical knowledge, for example knowledge of how to give injections, take blood pressures, deal with aggressive people, manage caseloads and so on.

Within the nursing domain, the question of whether there are distinct types of knowledge has been brought to prominence largely by the work of Patricia Benner (1984). Her work has prompted consideration of the distinction between propositional knowledge and practical knowledge. This same distinction can be cast in either of the following ways:

- As a distinction between knowing how and knowing that.
- As a distinction between theoretical and practical knowledge.
- As a distinction between intellectual and bodily knowledge. And lastly
- in Heidegger's (1962) hands, as a distinction between 'the ready-to-hand' (practical knowing) and 'the present-at-hand' (theoretical knowing).

In the Western philosophical tradition, due largely to the influence of Plato (for example *The Republic, Bk. VI*), the senses and the body have been viewed mainly as obstacles to the obtaining of knowledge. With a few exceptions, it has standardly been thought that reason only is that faculty of humans capable of obtaining knowledge, and that it is solely through the use of reason that knowledge is acquired. Hence, a model of knowledge follows in which it is held that knowledge consists in the apprehension, by the faculty of reason, of truths. Moreover, these truths are held to be in propositional form. So a person knows that something *p* is the case by standing in a particular kind of mental relation to a proposition *p*. Thus all knowledge, it is held, is 'knowledge that', equivalently, propositional knowledge. (This is the case even for philosophers within the 'empiricist' tradition.)

When it is applied to the question of what it is to know how to perform actions, such as giving an injection, or playing a piano, the view that all knowledge is propositional suggests that each component or 'step' of the relevant action has an equivalent proposition. This is then mentally 'grasped' by the actor and leads to the relevant step in the series of acts which completes the larger act. So on this model, giving an injection will involve the assumption that the task as a whole is composed of smaller, discrete steps for each of which there will be an equivalent mental 'proposition'. As the actor proceeds through the task he inwardly scans these propositions, rather like a mental instruction manual. What distinguishes the person who can perform the task (the expert) from one who cannot (the novice) is that the former has this internal manual and the latter has not.

This model of what is involved in the performance of skilled action fosters at least two assumptions. First, that there is a sharp distinction to be drawn between theory and practice. This should be evident in the gloss of the model just provided: one applies the 'theory', that is, one's knowledge of the mental propositions, to the practical task one is engaged in. The second assumption is that theory precedes practice (Ryle, 1949, p. 30; Benner and Wrubel, 1989, Chapter 2; Dreyfus, 1994, p. vii). This should be evident from the example just given: before being able to give an injection, one needs to learn and mentally 'store' the relevant series of instructions (for example, 1. Pick up the syringe, 2. Pick up the ampoule... and so on).

This model of practical knowing has been subjected to attack by Gilbert Ryle (1949, Chapter 2), and his work is one of the key sources in the attempt to establish that not all knowing is propositional in nature. In making his case Ryle makes a number of arguments, but two in particular are relevant for our purposes. The first runs thus (Ryle's term for the view that all knowledge is propositional is the 'intellectualist model'.)

Ryle suggests that apprehending/grasping/considering mental propositions is itself an activity. So, it seems reasonable to ask on what further set of propositions this activity is founded? Ryle points out that it is not possible for this supposed relationship between activities and propositions to go on indefinitely; in other words the 'intellectualist' position leads to an infinite regress. At some point, since we manifestly do act and think, we must simply act without its being the case that our actions are prompted by consideration of an 'inner', mental proposition.

Second, Ryle notes that there seems a clear sense in which practice is prior to theory. For example, the development of logic (theory of argumentation) is posterior to the presenting of arguments. Similarly, theories of nursing follow from the practice of nursing. Hence, such actions cannot be theory driven (that is, on the supposition that any set of mental propositions which generated nursing actions constituted a theory).

And, Ryle makes the following important observation: mere knowledge of a relevant set of propositions (for example a theory) is not sufficient for knowing how to perform a particular activity. One might be able to recite all the steps involved in giving an injection yet still be unable to give one. One might have no hands, or one might simply not yet have acquired the dexterity and familiarity with the relevant implements – the syringe, the ampoule – in order to draw up the required amount of the drug to be injected. It seems possible to advance innumerable other examples of this kind – for example regarding counselling, or managing a busy ward, or, away from the health care context, swimming, or cycling and so on.

These last considerations form a key part of Ryle's case against the intellectualist position according to which, as we have seen, the performance of actions requires mental scanning of inner propositions.

Moreover, Ryle draws attention to the differences in priority accorded to knowing how and knowing that respectively. For example, being able to recite the rules of chess is not sufficient for being able to play chess. So here, 'knowing that' (that is, knowing the rules of chess) does not imply that one can play chess. And if a person could play chess but not recite the rules it would still be allowed that the person was able to play chess. Hence, being able to recite the rules is not even a necessary condition of being able to play chess.

Thus Ryle seems to show that possession of 'knowledge that' is not a necessary condition of 'knowing how' (since a person may be able to play chess without being able to recite the rules), nor is 'knowing that' a sufficient condition of 'knowing how' (since the real test of whether a person can play lies in his performance).

So Ryle seems to show that knowing how need not be underpinned by knowing that, and to strongly suggest that these two types of knowledge are distinct. Further, Ryle does this by recruiting the kind of example which seems most suited to support the intellectualist case (that is, the case of playing chess).

A further interesting objection to the intellectualist account of practical knowledge is made by Merleau-Ponty (1962). This is that according to the intellectualist position, skill acquisition – such as that involved in playing chess – seems to proceed along the lines described above (insofar as it is thought to involve the learning of propositions which correspond to each step in the relevant task). But Merleau-Ponty argues that complex tasks are not simply amalgams or conjunctions of simpler tasks. He suggests, plausibly, that the components of a complex task are related in such a way that the sense or meaning of the component task is not independent of the complete task. Hence, playing a tune on an organ does not consist simply in performing each individual note. Rather, the significance of the individual notes is bound to the overall context – the performance, or at least the particular musical passage – as a whole (for example 1962, pp. 142–3). Merleau-Ponty provides the instructive example of typing in this context; the typist, he suggests, has 'knowledge in the hands' (1962, p. 144).

This quote is significant in that it gestures to a positive account of practical knowledge such that it is knowledge actually possessed by the body. This view conflicts radically with the Platonic one referred to earlier in which only minds can 'possess' knowledge.

So on the alternative, Merleau-Pontian view, the fluid movements of the musician, the footballer and the tennis player all manifest 'bodily' knowledge. And, with reference to the nursing context, the performance of complex motor tasks (for example giving injections again) can also be seen as exemplifications of bodily knowledge (for example Benner and Wrubel, 1989, pp. 42–5).

The fluidity of movement associated with expert performance of motor tasks is one of the features which helps to distinguish the novice from the expert performer; the novice, it may be said, has yet to acquire bodily knowledge.

In explanation of bodily knowledge, this is said to derive from 'bodily intentionality' (see, for example, Merleau-Ponty, 1962, p. 130; Benner and Wrubel, 1989, p. 76; Hammond et al., 1991, p. 180). To expand on this a little: We heard that according to the intellectualist story, the performance of (say) motor tasks involves reflection on mental propositions. But on this alternative line, the body itself 'represents' motor (and other) tasks. Hence, when one practices a complex sequence of movements which constitute the performance of a task, one's body is 'gearing in' to the task and intentionality or 'representation' of the task is acquired by the body. As Hammond et al. (1991, p. 180) put it:

> In performing such actions, one's body is not to be seen as guided by an intentional consciousness which exists independently of it: the intentionality instead belongs to the body itself...

So bodily 'intentionality' involves the representation of a task by the body. It is not a mental representation of the kind which is claimed in the intellectualist account of skilled motor performances (that is, in the 'mental instruction manual' model). It is such 'bodily intentionality' that the expert performer of a task has acquired but which the novice is still attempting to acquire.

It was mentioned earlier that the phenomenon of bodily knowledge has been thought to have particular relevance to practice disciplines such as nursing. This is in part due to the fact that nursing practice involves the performance of a range of motor skills – for example in handling medical instruments, taking blood pressures, giving injections and so on. But it should be borne in mind that bodily knowledge can be invoked to help highlight and explain a much broader range of skills than simply motor skills.

Benner and Wrubel point out that a wide range of phenomena which seem central to nursing involve bodily knowledge in a much more general sense than that invoked in the carrying out of motor tasks. For example, all the following kinds of actions can plausibly be claimed to manifest bodily knowledge: the performance of gestures by nurses, their responses to gestures from patients, the handling and coaxing of patients, moving patients, interpreting their expressions, touching patients, the posture of nurses and so on.

Having now set out the distinction between propositional and practical knowledge, it is worth pausing to consider just what can be concluded from acceptance of it.

First, the point that practice is *temporally* prior to theory, for example in nursing, does not show there to be no room for theory in nursing. All that is shown is that practice precedes theory. Therefore, second, even if practical knowledge is what is most central to nursing – since it is a practical discipline – it does not follow that there is no place for propositional knowledge. Clearly, in any plausible position on the kinds of information necessary for nursing some of this must be descriptive, for example relating to human physiology and so on.

Third, Ryle makes the point that, for example in chess playing, what matters ultimately is the performance. Thus even if a player proved incapable of listing the rules of chess, the question of whether or not he could play chess would be resolved by evaluating his performances. Ryle envisages the possibility that a player could be a competent chess player but not able to indicate descriptively that he knows the rules of chess.

It must be wondered whether a comparable example would be possible in the nursing context. Set aside the practical difficulties in considering whether a person could satisfy examination requirements and so on. Could a person function as a nurse and be incapable of relating, at least in part, descriptively what they do? It seems to me they could not. The reason is that being accountable is a necessary requirement of professional nursing practice, and this requires the possibility of giving reasons for actions, and has no parallel in Ryle's chess example.

Given the presumption, noted earlier, against the idea of bodily knowledge, and the fact that its legitimacy is somewhat taken for granted within nursing scholarship it may be worth considering briefly three objections to the legitimacy of such knowledge. As will be shown, each can be responded to.

Problems (and defences) concerning the idea of bodily knowledge

Hamlyn's distinction

Hamlyn suggests that a distinction should be made between knowing how to do something, and merely being able to do it. The former he suggests can properly be characterised as knowledge, but the latter cannot. Hence, Hamlyn holds: '"Knowing how" is knowledge of a technique...' (1970, p. 104). So 'know how' or what we have been describing as bodily knowledge properly describes what we might term skilled behaviours only. Thus, playing a musical instrument, or the other kinds of motor tasks mentioned earlier count as knowledge for Hamlyn because they involve some learning of a technique. Bodily movements such as moving one's fingers, or hands would not count as knowledge for Hamlyn – for the same reason. Hence, he says that it would 'seem strange to say that I know how to flex my muscles' (ibid.).

Evidently, Hamlyn wishes to restrict the term 'knowledge' to activities which require some degree of learning and practice. So voluntary movements of limbs, flexing of muscles and so on do not count as knowledge since they do not, so Hamlyn seems to assume, involve the learning of a technique.

However, this is precisely what is denied, with some plausibility, by Merleau-Ponty (1962). The neonate's early months are spent in pursuit of the acquisition of techniques such as flexing muscles, or as it was put earlier, 'gearing in' to the world. Similarly, following prolonged injury to a limb one has to re-learn to use it again, to coordinate its movements with the rest of one's body (see Sacks, 1984). So the challenge to the notion of bodily knowledge posed by Hamlyn's distinction can be repulsed.

A Wittgensteinian objection

The scope of bodily knowledge, it was suggested above, includes at least knowledge of motor tasks, and more general knowledge relating to posture, gesture, speech (for example tone of voice), mode of physical contact with others, and so on. Knowledge of the locations of one's own limbs, or knowledge of the sensations which one is currently experiencing – bodily knowledge in a, perhaps, more conventional sense of that term has not been referred to.

A point made by Wittgenstein concerning claims to know runs as follows. He suggests that knowledge claims are legitimate only in contexts where there is a possibility that one can be mistaken (for example 1953, p. 221, 1975). Since one cannot be mistaken about the location of one's limbs, or whether or not one is (say) in pain, it makes no sense to claim to know any of these things.

Of course, there are some medical conditions – agnosias – in which people precisely are unable to judge the locations of their limbs (Sacks, 1984) and so in such cases one can envisage situations in which legitimate claims to know are possible on Wittgenstein's criterion. However, it should be said that for most of us our predicament does not resemble that of the agnosic and so, if we accept Wittgenstein's move, claims to know locations of our limbs and our sensations seem vulnerable to this line of criticism.

In defence of the idea of bodily knowledge as it applies to the kind of practical knowledge involved in nursing, against Wittgenstein, the idea of knowledge does seem applicable. For example, there is a clear difference between the fumbling manipulation of a syringe manifested by a novice nurse, and the smoothly executed movements of the more experienced nurse. When the novice acquires the level of skill displayed by the expert it seems reasonable to say the novice has learned how to perform this skill, or that he has progressed from not knowing how to do it, to knowing how to do it.

So the Wittgensteinian point may apply legitimately to claims to know the locations of one's limbs and so on (agnosias apart), but it can be resisted in its applicability to bodily knowledge per se.

A 'logical' objection

In his account of knowledge and belief, Luper-Foy (1992, p. 234) refers to an 'entailment thesis' such that

> knowledge entails belief, so that I cannot know that such and such is the case unless I believe that such and such is the case (see also, Hamlyn, 1970, p. 101).

This seems relatively unproblematic in cases of propositional knowledge. If I know that Swansea is west of Cardiff it seems reasonable to suppose that I also believe this. However, in bodily knowing it is less clear that such an entailment thesis applies. For example, playing the piano cannot simply amount to knowledge of a sequence of 'beliefs that...' given what was argued earlier concerning the distinction between knowing that and knowing how.

So it seems either that the entailment thesis would have to be revised in order to accommodate bodily knowledge; or, if the entailment thesis is to be held as a necessary condition of knowledge, it would have to be conceded that bodily knowledge is not knowledge. Alternatively, it can be proposed that the entailment thesis applies only to propositional knowledge and not to practical knowledge. And, given our scepticism about the idea of knowledge in general, it is an option to concede that bodily knowledge is not in fact knowledge but some weaker epistemic property. Either of these seem reasonable responses.

Before moving on now to apply these points to the discussion of the works of Carper and Benner, four final points need to be made.

First, an attribution of practical knowledge must be relative to some specific task, or more broadly, domain. Thus, it would not be very informative to say a person has practical knowledge. For this to be other than empty, the attribution would need to be narrowed down to a specific task, for example mending punctures, or to some domain of expertise, say, within the domain of nursing, engineering or some other area requiring practical knowledge.

Second, a plausible necessary condition for the attribution to a person of practical knowledge must be that they can successfully perform that task. This is the case whether the attribution is task- or domain-specific. Legitimately to ascribe to a person practical knowledge in relation to a specific type of task requires, at least, that they can standardly perform that task. And legitimate ascription to a person of domain specific practical knowledge – for example that necessary to be a good nurse – requires that they can meet the standards considered appropriate for that domain.

Third, given the role of evidence in relation to propositional knowledge, is there a similar role for evidence in relation to practical knowledge? One possibility would involve a focus upon the question of whether the ends of the action were achieved. Thus evidence that a person had practical knowledge to perform tasks needs to take into account success in achieving that task. More generally, evidence that a person has domain-specific practical know-how would require successful performance of their specific role within that domain. Thus within nursing it would require meeting the ends of nursing as these were currently conceived.

Finally, given the difference between knowledge and belief within the domain of propositional knowledge, one wonders if a similar difference can be identified within the field of practical knowledge. In the propositional domain, knowledge matches how the world happens to be, how it is. Knowledge in this field aims at description, and necessarily successfully describes; the success of belief in describing accurately is contingent only (since beliefs may be false). Within the practical domain it can be claimed that practical knowledge aims at and meets the relevant practical ends aimed at. 'Practical belief', as it were, is less successful in terms of meeting the practical ends aimed at.

It should be conceded that this is not a distinction immune from rigorous criticism. For even a possessor of practical knowledge might occasionally fail to reach the end aimed at. Thus, as with the propositional domain, it may be best to allow that only practical belief is possible, and that this comes in varying degrees of strength. The expert possesses strong 'practical belief', fallible but rarely missing its aim. The novice possesses only weak 'practical belief', frequently missing its aim.

So, we began this chapter by considering just why the topic of knowledge is considered central to nursing. We then moved on to discuss propositional knowledge. The conclusion reached is that knowledge claims are essentially revisable. We must be prepared for the possibility that beliefs we currently take to be true might, nonetheless, turn out to be mistaken. Thus an attitude of modesty is warranted in relation to what we currently take to be known.

Our discussion of practical knowledge involved a defence of the distinction between practical and propositional knowledge, and also a defence of the idea of bodily knowledge from some other philosophical sources. We saw, lastly, that a distinction within the realm of practical knowledge is possible which 'parallels', in some respects, that between propositional knowledge and belief. Whereas propositional knowledge 'aims at' truth, so to speak, practical knowing 'aims at' successful performance of the relevant skill or task.

Having discussed both propositional and practical knowledge, we can now move on to discuss two landmark contributions to the subject of nursing knowledge. These are from Carper and Benner respectively.

3 Nursing knowledge (ii): Carper and Benner on knowledge

We now continue our enquiry within the realm of epistemology by looking first at an important paper by Carper. We then turn to discuss Benner's work on nursing knowledge specifically as presented in her 1984 book From Novice to Expert (FNE). *As noted in Chapter 1, we might locate these discussions within both 'philosophical presuppositions' and 'scholarship' strands of philosophy of nursing. The chapter ends with a more general discussion of the very idea of nursing knowledge.*

Carper's 'Fundamental Patterns of Knowing in Nursing' (1978) (*FPKN*)

Carper's paper *FPKN* is an extremely influential contribution to discussions of knowledge within the nursing canon. It forms the standard reference point for discussions of knowledge within nursing (see for example McKenna, 1997). The work done in the paper has been applied to structure specific genres of nursing research (for example reflective practice, see Johns, 1995). Its influence and stature within the nursing canon demand that we have a close look at Carper's paper since if it has flaws there is a worry that these may have been passed down within nursing scholarship over the past 20 years.

In the paper Carper begins by asserting the importance of 'critical attention to the question of what it means to know' (*FPKN*, p. 13) (henceforth within this chapter, references in page numbers only refer to this paper). This clearly seems crucial in a paper concerned to explicate knowledge 'fundamental' to nursing. She then famously identifies 'Four fundamental patterns of knowing' within nursing (pp. 13–14). These four patterns are said to comprise the 'kinds of knowledge [that] are held to be of most value in the discipline of nursing' (p. 13). The four patterns Carper identifies are 'empirics', 'esthetics', 'personal knowledge', and 'ethics' (pp. 14–20). I will run very briefly through each of these, and close the discussion of Carper by signalling some fairly fundamental shortcomings in her paper. Perhaps alarmingly, these normally pass unnoticed within nursing literature, and it will be an aim of this discussion to at least try to clarify Carper's own task within *FPKN*.

It will be suggested here that Carper's own paper exemplifies the need for 'critical attention to the question of what it means to know'; in fact, as will be seen below, the expression 'patterns of knowing' itself seems needlessly obscure and confusing.

The first pattern of knowing identified by Carper is: 'Empirics: the science of nursing' (p. 14). Her discussion of this focuses on empirical knowledge, specifically that drawn from empirical sciences related to nursing, for example physiology and pathology (p. 15).

Discussion of this pattern concludes, 'Thus the first fundamental pattern of knowing is empirical, factual, descriptive... It is exemplary, discursively formulated and publicly verifiable' (p. 15). So this pattern relates to the empirical knowledge considered necessary in order to nurse. It is 'empirical' in that it is acquired by deployment of the senses, by empirical investigation into, for example, the human body. It is considered 'factual' by Carper, presumably on the grounds that it is knowledge rather than mere belief. It is 'descriptive' in the sense that it describes regions of the world, for example, relevantly for nursing, the workings of the human body. The reference to verifiability is related to the descriptive nature of empirical claims: typically, such claims are open to scrutiny from the third person perspective (though of course some are not, for example relating to events in the distant past).

Carper's second pattern is 'esthetics: the art of nursing' (p. 16). She suggests that this can be usefully contrasted with scientific modes of thinking. Art is described as 'expressive' and not merely 'formal or descriptive' in the way that science is (p. 16). Moreover, aesthetic experiences resist description in language: 'The knowledge gained by subjective acquaintance, the direct feeling of experience, defies discursive formulation' (p. 16). This is held to be in contrast to empirical knowledge, which as seen, can be 'discursively formulated' (p. 15).

Carper is usually taken to be referring to practical knowing here (see for example McKenna, 1997, p. 41). As she indicates, this is acquired from performance of practical tasks, the 'feeling of experience' – how it feels to perform these, and so on. Thus, for example, learning how to give an injection or use a sphygmomanometer requires developing a feel for such instruments and their proper use. It takes time and familiarity with them to become able to use them appropriately smoothly (that is, to acquire the appropriate bodily intentionality).

It is likely that Carper coins the term 'esthetic' knowing in this context due to the view that practical knowledge involves mastery of an 'art'. Thus it may be said that a skilled nurse is one whose actions manifest mastery of 'the art of nursing'. Given this, and that 'aesthetics' involves the enquiry into the properties manifested by works of art (beauty, ugliness, symmetry and so on), it may then be concluded with Carper that the art of nursing involves aesthetic knowing.

Carper's summary of this pattern runs thus:

> The esthetic pattern of knowing in nursing involves the perception of abstracted particulars as distinguished from the recognition of abstracted universals (p. 18).

This sounds very different from practical knowing, but can be taken as claiming that the aesthetic pattern of knowing involves perception of particular patients as opposed simply to 'the patient' considered in the abstract.

So this pattern involves knowledge of particular patients, the kind of appreciation of their predicament which comes from experience and sensitivity. And in defence of Carper, since this kind of sensitivity is something which may be a form of practical knowing, there need not be a tension between her concluding remarks about this pattern of knowing and the interpretation of it as a form of practical knowing.

The third pattern is 'The component of personal knowledge' (p. 18). For Carper this is 'the most essential to understanding the meaning of health in terms of individual well-being' (p. 18). Further, 'Personal knowledge is concerned with the knowing, encountering and actualizing of the concrete, individual self' (p. 18). Roughly speaking, the suggestion here is that in order to nurse others, it is necessary to know oneself. As she states, 'personal knowing extends not only to other selves but also to relations with one's own self (p. 18). Indeed, for Carper, it seems that one can only understand what health may be for someone else, if one has personal knowledge. Not only is personal knowledge necessary to help patients become healthy, it is necessary even to encounter another self.

Carper's fourth pattern of knowing in nursing is 'Ethics: the moral component' (p. 20). 'The ethical pattern of knowing in nursing requires an understanding of different philosophical positions regarding... different ethical frameworks...' (p. 21). As may be anticipated, in the light of the moral dimension of nursing practice, Carper considers sensitivity to this crucial. But further, Carper suggests that more than mere sensitivity to this moral dimension is necessary. An 'understanding' of different moral theories and perspectives within ethics is also necessary. Presumably it is envisaged that such understanding will help practitioners in their moral reasoning in the practical moral problems which they inevitably face.

With regard to all four patterns, Carper suggests: 'Each pattern may be conceived as necessary for achieving mastery in the discipline [of nursing]' (pp. 21–2).

> Nursing thus depends on the scientific knowledge of human behavior in health and in illness, the esthetic perception of significant human experiences, a personal understanding of the unique individuality of the self and the capacity to make choices within concrete situations involving particular moral judgments (p. 22).

Carper also adds: 'all knowledge is subject to change and revision' (p. 22).

Critique of Carper's FPKN

Having set out some of the claims within *FPKN* let us now consider some criticisms.

A first, and basic point concerns the distinction between knowledge and belief. As seen earlier, this is plainly a fundamental distinction, reflecting crucial differences in the relations of these to truth, and consequently in the level of cognitive security which can be rested upon a claim.

Given the distinction between knowledge and belief, and the nature of our discussion of it, it is evident that the points which Carper makes, *very strictly speaking*, should be taken to apply at the level of belief and not knowledge. Carper's claim that 'all knowledge is subject to change' (p. 22) shows this. For as we saw above, on the model of knowledge outlined earlier, if a claim is later shown to be false then it cannot be said to have been known, only believed.

Our earlier discussion of the concept of knowledge has other ramifications also for the claims of Carper and we can now begin to discuss these.

Consider the four realms of knowledge-claims which Carper identifies: empirics, aesthetics, personal knowledge and ethics.

With regard to empirics, our Quinean view suggests no scientific statement is immune from revision. Given this, the empirical domain as Carper conceives of this cannot be known about. For knowledge requires the truth of what is known, and since following Quine, no statement is immune from revision, no empirical claim can be known, only believed.

It is important to bear in mind that it does not follow from this that all such beliefs stand on the same footing. As was stressed in the discussion of Quine's position, knowledge claims for which good evidence can be produced are to be favoured over those unsupported by evidence – at least within this domain (in addition to other 'virtues' which can be employed to assess claims). Thus rejection of the view that there can be knowledge of the function of the human body is consistent with there being some claims which are more plausible than others. The claim that human beings have hearts is more plausible than the claim that they do not; as is the claim that hearts have four chambers. But however certain we currently feel about these claims, it is conceivable they be revised at some later date. Lest this possibility itself seems inconceivable, try to imagine how contrary to common sense it must have been to have been informed that the Earth is not, in fact, stationary but is orbiting the Sun at thousands of miles per hour. Yet this (currently) passes as one of our most cherished scientific views about the nature of the Earth.

These considerations show that Carper's empirical 'pattern of knowing' ought not to be taken to involve empirical knowledge. Rather, at least on one interpretation of what a 'pattern of knowing' is, it concerns beliefs about empirical matters.

In relation to the aesthetic domain, it should be said that the whole idea of evidence appears problematic here. Empirical claims such as those relating to the function of the human body can be tested and either supported or not. Here there is a tribunal of evidence which can be appealed to in order to resolve disputes. But what would count as evidence that one work of art is 'better than' another? Counting heads has never been a good way to determine whether a work of art is a classic or a dud. In any case, why should the popularity of a work of art count in its favour and not against it? This seems an especially pertinent point in relation to, say, popular works in music or fiction. The aesthetic status accorded to such works by art critics generally fails to match their popular appeal. So given the problems in identifying a tribunal which can be appealed to in disputes regarding the worth of works of art, the idea of aesthetic knowing seems problematic.

Matters are further complicated by the fact that Carper's recruitment of the term 'aesthetics' may not even be appropriate. The reason is that Carper seems to be discussing practical knowledge within the discussion of the aesthetic pattern of knowing. As noted earlier, the realm of aesthetics (at least in modern post-17th-century usage) is the realm of the enquiry into aesthetic properties, notably that of beauty, the kind of properties exemplified by works of art (paintings, sculptures, music, literature and so on). Her concern is with the 'art' of nursing and there are good grounds to suppose questions of aesthetics to be peripheral to this domain. For what matters in nursing is whether the nurse nurses properly, and this need not amount to behaving 'beautifully' or even 'gracefully'. (See Chapter 9 below, plus de Raeve, 1998, and Wainwright, 1999, for more on this issue.)

According to Carper's own official characterisation of the aesthetic domain it 'defies discursive formulation' (p. 16). Given this, one might suppose it to be highly problematic to apply the notion of evidence to it.

One strategy, however, to try to recover the idea of knowledge in relation to the 'art of nursing', is as follows. Suppose aesthetic knowing is understood as relating to the performance of nursing skills – if it is aligned with practical knowing – then 'evidence' might be cashed out by reference to the relationship between nursing actions, and the ends aimed at. Hence, even if we could not explain why one nurse was skilled at defusing dangerously aggressive episodes, while another nurse was less successful in attempts to do so, it would be evident that one nurse was more successful than another in such attempts.

Due to the difficulty in specifying – discursively formulating – aesthetic knowing, it would not be possible to describe in detail what it is that one nurse possesses and the other lacks. But it would be possible to state the 'success rates' of the two nurses in meeting the ends of nursing, in some specific context. So perhaps the idea of evidence can apply at some level here, in terms of the success or otherwise at meeting the ends of nursing.

It should be stressed, however, that there are serious grounds to criticise Carper's claims in relation to this pattern of knowing. She seems to conflate the ideas of art and skilled performance of a craft. From the fact that works of art necessarily have aesthetic properties, she concludes erroneously that skilled performance of nursing actions similarly must possess such properties. It is suggested here that such properties are at most contingent, accidental features of nursing actions. As suggested above, surely what matters most is whether or not nursing acts meet the ends of nursing.

What of Carper's discussion of personal knowledge? This includes having knowledge of the kind of person one is. Minimally, this might be taken to involve knowledge of one's values, and one's strengths and weaknesses. Then, it may be claimed, it is necessary to know this much about oneself in order properly to nurse others.

Again, however, there seem serious difficulties here for Carper. Let us distinguish two claims:

- that self-knowledge is unproblematic and certainly possible; and
- that self-knowledge is necessary for (good) nursing practice

(recall that Carper thinks it is: 'each pattern may be conceived as necessary...' (p. 21)).

With regard to the first of these claims, it seems dubious to claim that one knows oneself. I have views about what my values are, and about what my strengths and weaknesses are, but it doesn't follow that I know what these are. Relatedly, Freud's work on the unconscious suggests that our real motivations are not transparent to us. These reflections do not, of course, call into question the very idea of self-knowledge, but they show it to be fairly problematic.

A further indication of its problems arises when it is considered how it could be shown that a person, in fact, has personal knowledge. Can one claim to know that one is a good person, say? Certainly more would be required in order to answer this than one's own opinion. Hence, necessarily, there is a role for considerations gleaned from persons other than the person concerned. It follows from this that a gap is always possible between what is claimed to be known and the evidence appealed to – given the sceptical worries rehearsed earlier. So the idea of personal knowledge also seems problematic, at least as problematic as the idea of empirical knowledge.

With regard to the second claim identified above, here also it seems to me Carper's line is dubious. In saying that personal knowledge is necessary for (good) nursing practice, Carper is claiming that it is required for practice in all areas of nursing. Assessment of this question is not helped by the ambiguity surrounding the idea of personal knowledge, but the following query seems a reasonable one. For example, one might argue there is a place for personal knowledge in areas of nursing such as psychiatry, but what of contexts in which very little personal contact need take place, such as intensive care nursing, accident and emergency, and public health nursing?

Moreover, given the reference to Freudian views concerning the extent of our self-knowledge, it may actually be an advantage to lack self-knowledge. For example, suppose a nurse thinks of himself as a caring person who nurses for largely altruistic reasons. Suppose his work is highly valued by patients and colleagues. After a period of psychoanalysis the nurse comes to realise that his 'real' motivations for becoming a nurse are self- rather than other-oriented. This affects his performance as a nurse, he puts less hours in and is more likely to place his own needs above those of his patients – having recognised that this accords with the desires of his 'real' self. Colleagues and patients notice this difference in the nurse and, frankly, prefer the nurse when he lacked the self-knowledge acquired during analysis. If accepted, this vignette calls into question the view, suggested by Carper, that the more self-knowledge one has, the better nurse one will be.

Consider now the ethical pattern of knowing. As before, two queries arise immediately with the idea of knowledge of moral matters. One concerns the possibility of moral knowledge, as knowledge. The other concerns the peculiar dimension of problems in virtue of which they are moral rather than empirical problems.

With regard to the first question, plainly, if knowledge per se is unattainable, so too will moral knowledge be. So the most one can speak of here are more and less plausible beliefs about moral matters. In relation to the second question, the problem of resolving disputes about moral questions is due to an extra layer of complexity which is not present in disputes concerning empirical matters. This extra layer can be illustrated thus: it can be agreed that a patient has a cancerous tumour. There are standard empirically established tests in order to determine this. So in this example there is agreement about the patient's physical condition, and this is based upon agreed procedures concerning how this can be determined. However, this agreement at the level of empirical matters need not entail agreement at the level of the moral dimension of the situation. One health care professional may judge that the patient should be given the information about the cancerous tumour, another may judge that he should not. The point here is that the means available to settle any dispute concerning empirical questions, seem not to be available in order to settle any moral dispute – for example, concerning whether or not the patient should be given the information. Thus the possibility of moral knowledge appears doubly imperilled: first due to the scepticism regarding the possibility of there being any knowledge, and second due to the apparent difference between the moral and empirical domains.

It should be stressed once again here that the position just sketched does not entail that all beliefs about moral matters stand on an equal footing. Moral judgements, like other types of judgement, can be supported by reasons and these can be good or bad, relevant or irrelevant and so on. So denying there can be moral knowledge need not entail moral subjectivism (the view that all beliefs about moral matters are equally legitimate). It is plain, however, that none of these issues is evident in Carper's discussion and so once more her account of the four patterns appears vulnerable to criticism.

Having now discussed each of the four patterns of knowing she identifies we can turn now to consider the question of what a pattern of knowing actually is. Carper's paper seems to me to be ambiguous and to suggest two ways of answering this question.

The first is that Carper is pointing to four *sources* of knowledge; or, put another way, to four ways in which phenomena can be known. On this reading of Carper, the senses (presumably) would be the sources of our empirical information, an equivalent aesthetic sense would be the source of aesthetic beliefs, and so on for the other two patterns.

This interpretation raises several problems. First, surely, there is a clear and important distinction between the sources of knowledge and knowledge itself. This is easily shown: to recall an example we used earlier, my sense of sight leads me to think railway lines converge, when of course they don't. Similarly, a stick looks bent when half immersed in water; again, it does not follow from this that it is bent; and so on, and so on. Senses provide us with information, but it does not follow from this that the information is always accurate. (Think also of examples of illusory figures from cognitive psychology, such as the Muller-Lyer illusion, and so on.)

So there is a clear difference between sources of knowledge and knowledge itself. The senses lead us to acquire and develop beliefs, some of which are barely credible (for example hallucinations), some of which are plausible. Carper's discussion seems to conflate these two importantly different aspects of human experience.

We have just discussed the interpretation of Carper's patterns of knowing as sources of knowledge with reference to the empirical pattern, and seen that this is very problematic. It may also be problematic in relation to the aesthetic and ethical patterns. Take the first of these. Objects of aesthetic appreciation are also empirical objects – objects the existence of which we recognise due to the information they reflect into our retinas, or other receptors of sensory information such as the skin, or the tongue. Thus I become visually aware of a painting when patterns of light from it are reflected into my retina. So any aesthetic object is also an empirical object. It follows that the empirical and aesthetic patterns of knowing coincide. For in coming to know an object in terms of its aesthetic properties I also come to know it in terms of its empirical properties.

In response to this point, it is open to Carper to suggest that the aesthetic properties exemplified by objects are over and above their empirical ones, and that the recognition of this extra 'layer' of properties amounts to an aesthetic pattern of knowing. Such a pattern, thus construed, amounts to what can be termed a 'sensibility', a capacity to recognise the aesthetic dimension of experience. It should be stressed again, however, that the presence of this sensibility is not sufficient for the possession of aesthetic knowledge.

A similar story can be told in relation to the ethical pattern of knowing. Situations which exhibit a moral dimension will inevitably also exemplify empirical properties. Hence seeing a person strike another inevitably involves the perception of empirical phenomena. As with the aesthetic pattern, it can be allowed that the moral dimension of empirical phenomena is something over and above the empirical dimension. And it can be allowed that a moral sensibility is necessary in order to recognise the moral dimension of human experience. Finally, once more, it needs to be stressed that none of this shows such a pattern to deliver knowledge, only belief.

Thus, there seem serious problems with the construal of patterns of knowing as *sources* of knowledge.

I have not yet mentioned personal knowledge since here there does seem a clear sense in which one has a source of information about one's own thoughts and feelings which differs importantly from others' access to this information. One might be in company with others feeling awful but looking and behaving cheerfully. There seems something privileged in this kind of access which one uniquely has to one's feelings and thoughts (which is not to allow that this access necessarily brings personal knowledge). (See, for example, Alston, 1971.) So perhaps it is in relation to personal knowing that the construal of a pattern of knowing as a source of knowledge is most promising.

The second interpretation of what Carper means by her expression 'pattern of knowing' is as follows. A fairly simplistic way to read Carper's term is that it refers to types or classes of knowledge claims. Thus, on this reading she should simply be taken to be pointing to four types of knowledge which seem important to nursing: scientific, aesthetic, moral and personal. As we have seen, it is very problematic to claim that any of these types of knowledge do in fact amount to knowledge, but let us construe them as areas of knowledge claims. So in nursing it is important to be aware of relevant scientific knowledge claims, for example relating to biology and chemistry. This seems uncontroversial and plausible.

But as pointed out earlier, the idea even of knowledge claims in relation to the aesthetic domain is very problematic. Worse, it is far from clear that Carper is in fact suggesting that awareness of knowledge claims in the domain of aesthetics is central to nursing. As noted earlier, her discussion of aesthetic knowing suffers from a crippling ambiguity. It is most plausibly read as relating to the kinds of practical skills one needs in order to nurse. Aesthetics seems entirely peripheral to nursing. An interesting claim to the effect that aesthetics is central to nursing would have to show a necessary connection between that domain and the ends of nursing. But as suggested earlier, what matters most in nursing is whether or not the ends aimed at are obtained, not whether the means display aesthetic properties such as beauty and grace. (Recall our distinction in Chapter 1 between necessary and contingent truths.)

The moral domain, however, does seem central to nursing. The ends of nursing are moral ends and the acts which bring about those ends typically involve a moral dimension. Sensitivity to this dimension of nursing is vital. So Carper's position can be taken as one in which awareness of moral knowledge claims is important to proper practice.

Lastly, with regard to personal knowledge, this includes awareness of one's strengths and weaknesses, and for reasons given above, it seems controversial to me to regard this as necessary for proper nursing practice.

So, in criticism of Carper, it has been argued that she does not see the significance of the distinction between knowledge and belief. Nor does she seem to see that notions of aesthetic, moral and personal knowledge are problematic independently of the knowledge/belief issue. In addition, we were able to identify two ways of reading the expression 'pattern of knowing': as a source of knowledge, and as an area of knowledge claims relevant to nursing. This last sense was suggested here to be the more plausible way of construing Carper's expression. Thus her four patterns of knowing are best understood as four areas of knowledge claims relevant to nursing (though even here it remains problematic to see how knowledge claims in aesthetics can be relevant to nursing).

It might be complained that the reconstrual of claims relating to knowledge as claims about belief are simply examples of excessive nit-picking. However, consideration of some of the claims made by Benner in relation to expert practice can help to show the value of using the term 'knowledge' sparingly and strictly. To this task we now turn.

Benner on knowledge: (a) novice/expert; (b) intuition; (c) propositional and practical knowing

Next, I would like to give some indication of the nature of Benner's claims about knowledge. This will provide us with a further context within which to locate some of the philosophical worries raised in the previous chapter.

The discussion of Benner's work will focus on the following three main themes:

(a) the distinction between novices and experts;
(b) the concept of intuition; and
(c) the distinction between propositional and practical knowledge.

In her book *From Novice to Expert: Excellence and Power in Clinical Nursing Practice* (1984) (*FNE*) Benner sets out a specific view of the nature of the knowledge which skilled, 'expert' nurses possess and manifest in their practice. The position of the expert is of course contrasted with that of the novice. Following Dreyfus and Dreyfus (1980), Benner discerns five stages in the transition from novice to expert, these are: novice, advanced beginner, competent, proficient, and finally, expert.

It is not important for the discussion here to go through all these stages as Benner describes them. What is instructive about her discussion for our purposes is the opportunity it presents for an investigation into the nature of knowledge. Having done this, it will prove possible to have a clearer grasp of the position she endorses and its strengths and weaknesses.

The novice/expert distinction

Famously, Benner discusses the differences between expert and novice nurses. One important difference between these two groups relates to the way in which situations are viewed. Benner suggests 'the novice operates on abstract principles and formal models and theories' (1984, p. 193). Thus, consider a student nurse learning communication skills. He learns a (hypothetical) principle of 'postural echo' according to which when two people are communicating with each other they tend to adopt the same posture. So if one person is leaning forward to speak to the other, then that person will also lean forward, for example. Suppose the student is working in a mental health context with some anxious patients, which he wants to encourage to relax and to reduce their levels of anxiety. The student enters into a conversation with a particular patient, sitting beside him. At this stage in the situation, both are leaning forward in their chairs, the student is echoing the posture of the patient. The student then recalls the communication skills lecture and the general principle of postural echo. He then puts this into action by adopting a more relaxed seating position. The patient's posture also changes into the more relaxed position, thus echoing that of the student.

This example indicates the way a novice can put into practice an 'abstract principle' – in this case the principle of postural echo. The novice has to recognise a situation as one to which the principle can be applied, and then consciously to rehearse in his mind its application. He also notes the outcome of its application: which in this case was 'successful', confirming the principle.

The principle can be termed 'abstract' in the sense that, for novices learning about it in class (even if this involves role-play), they will not have encountered its concrete application in an actual clinical situation. To that extent the principle is an abstract one. The principle is also abstract in the sense that, as it is presented in the classroom setting, it relates to no specific patient or person that the novice has come across. Prior to its concrete application in the clinical context, the principle has no particularity: it generalises over patients in the abstract. Only when it is applied by the novice to a specific patient does the abstract principle acquire some particular content, some application to a specific patient with whom the novice has a clinical relationship.

All this contrasts with the performance of the expert nurse, 'expert human decision makers can get a gestalt of the situation...' (1984, p. xviii). The expert nurse 'perceives the situation as a whole, uses past concrete situations as paradigms, and moves to the accurate region of the problem without wasteful consideration of a large number of irrelevant options' (ibid., p. 3). And lastly, expert nurses develop 'global sets about patients', which involve a 'predisposition to act' (ibid., p. 7).

Thus if we consider again the same kind of situation which faced the student nurse. The expert nurse will have identified the patient as being anxious and will seek to do something about this. This may involve the 'principle of postural echo' described above, but at no stage will the expert nurse rehearse that principle or 'intentionally' apply it. The expert will have a 'set' which predisposes him to act in the appropriate therapeutic manner, which may in this example, to an observer, involve application of the postural echo principle. The expert's performance, however, does not involve conscious rehearsal of ways of reducing the anxiety of the patient. His past experience informs and guides his actions (ibid., p. 193). So the application of the principle is against a background of repeated applications of it in previous clinical situations. Some of these will include situations where the principle applied successfully, but it is likely that there were occasions when it failed. Experience in applying the principle thus makes available to the expert a range of data unavailable to the novice, and to the less sensitive practitioner. In the light of the expert's possession of this range of experience, Benner suggests 'the expert develops many perceptual distinctions that are not possible to learn or grasp conceptually' (ibid., p. 187). So this bank of experience undergone by the expert makes it possible for him to notice distinctions which the novice would miss, and which might account for those situations in which application of the 'principle' worked and those when it failed.

It should be added that, for Benner, the nature of expert practice cannot be set out in step-by-step fashion (1984, p. 42). For nursing is not 'procedural' but is 'holistic' (ibid.). In other words, echoing the earlier points regarding the differences between novice and expert perception of situations, the expert regards situations as a whole, the novice is forced to focus on specific aspects of situations. (Recall also Merleau-Ponty's claim regarding the holistic character of practical knowing.)

Before offering some comment on Benner's distinction between novice and expert, I'd like to draw attention to two further aspects of it. An interesting difference between the novice and the expert, introduced by Benner, concerns the idea of 'salience'. The suggestion here is that the expert, in monitoring the situation within a clinical environment, is able to home in on clinically salient areas of it. Thus, sticking with the example of the anxious patient, the novice may be unable to explain just why they interacted with that specific patient as opposed to another on the ward. By contrast, the expert's decision to interact with one patient as opposed to another can be explained by appeal to his sense of clinical salience developed over his period of nursing experience.

Related to the phenomenon of clinical salience, Benner discusses situations in which nurses appear to be able to predict sudden deterioration in a patient's condition. For example, a phenomenon termed the 'grey zone' is discussed (1984, p. 96). In this, 'patient changes were subtle and the margins of safety narrow' (ibid.). Also, Benner writes of 'vague hunches and global assessments that initially bypass critical analysis' (ibid., p. xviii); and further, 'Expert nurses often describe their perceptual abilities using phrases such as "gut feeling", a "sense of uneasiness", or a "feeling that things are not quite right"' (ibid., p. xviii). Such 'feelings' may relate to a patient's imminent heart failure or some other acute clinical episode.

The kind of phenomenon under discussion is one which many experienced nurses claim experience of. And it is fair to say that Benner's highlighting of this phenomenon has particular resonance for many nurses. Moreover, at least some of the features of expertise in nursing identified by Benner seem to involve this kind of judgement. A term which may be useful in order to focus our discussion of this phenomenon is that of intuition.

Intuition

Although Benner uses that term only rarely in *FNE* her position within that book is commonly taken to be one in which expert judgement derives from a special kind of intuition (for example English, 1993, p. 389; Cash, 1995). (It is worth noting that the term 'intuition' does not appear in the index of *FNE*, although there is a glossary entry for 'intuitive grasp'.) A question arises, of course, in relation to the nature of this intuition. As far as I can discern within *FNE*, in discussions of the kinds of situations such as those within the 'grey zone' Benner's writing (within *FNE*) sustains at least two interpretations, which differ importantly. The first interpretation is one in which no empirically available information prompts the expert's judgement that something is wrong with the patient. This interpretation appears supported by Benner's references to 'gut feelings' or 'a sense of uneasiness' (1984, p. xviii); and on the same page Benner seems to deny that such expert judgements need be based upon 'explicit signals' (p. xviii). One reasonable way to interpret these characterisations of expert judgement is that they are not based upon empirically available information. This interpretation, thus, accredits experts with a kind of mystical ability to foretell the future, if imprecisely, to the effect that '"something" is wrong with that patient'; or, less vaguely, 'that patient is about to erupt in temper'.

Although the text of *FNE* suggests the interpretation just given, other parts of it explicitly reject the assimilation of intuition with any kind of mystical power. Thus Benner's glossary definition of 'intuitive grasp' states 'this should not be confused with mysticism' (1984, p. 295). Also, Benner suggests experts are 'picking up on subtle changes...' (ibid., p. 100). So a second interpretation is available which allows that intuitive judgements are prompted by (presumably) empirically available information. The nature and subtlety of these cues is suggested in Benner's remark that 'expert human decision makers can get a gestalt of the situation...' (ibid., p. xviii). In other words, as mentioned above, they see a situation as a whole. Something within this ability to see situations as a whole renders the expert sensitive to phenomena unavailable to non-experts.

One explanation of just how the expert differs from the non-expert is this. It is reported that chess experts view the game in terms of complex patterns. Thus when asked to look at the current position of a game they proved able to recall the locations of 20–25 pieces. Non-experts by contrast could recall the positions of far fewer pieces. But when pieces were set on a board in random positions both experts and non-experts performed at the same level (reported in Haber and Hershenson, 1980).

These findings can be taken to suggest that experts think in terms of pattern recognition. Thus when viewing a patient, the pattern displayed by the 'data' is taken by the expert to signal imminent deterioration/aggression and so on.

Regardless of the precise mechanism of expert intuition, the main distinction for our purposes is between two positions on intuitive judgement. A first position is one in which intuition amounts to mysticism, where it is held there are no empirical signs upon which the expert implicitly relies in making clinical judgements. The second position is one in which the intuitive judgements of experts do rely upon some empirically available signs, however subtle. Although both these positions can be gleaned from a loose reading of *FNE*, it seems reasonable to accept that Benner's own position is closer to the second just described.

Let us now turn to a third key theme within *FNE*.

Practical and theoretical (propositional) knowledge

The distinction between 'practical and theoretical knowledge' (1984, p. 1) is central to appreciating the significance of Benner's work. As seen, the distinction has a fairly long history in philosophical discussions of knowledge (see Aristotle, *Ethics*, Bk. iv, Chapter 4) and it has received lengthy attention from some eminent 20th-century philosophers (Ryle, 1949; Polanyi, 1958; Heidegger, 1962).

As with Ryle, Benner rejects the view that all knowledge is propositional, and she supports the view that practical knowledge differs in kind from propositional knowledge. Further, again as with Ryle, Benner holds that possession of practical knowledge with regard to the performance of some activity A need not entail possession of propositional knowledge with respect to A. For Benner, possession of propositional knowledge is neither a necessary nor a sufficient condition of possession of practical knowledge. Moreover, practical knowledge of at least some types of practical activity cannot be fully specified in propositional terms.

An example which illustrates this nicely relates to the '"feel" of a contracted uterus' (1984, p. 5). It is reasonable to suppose there to be more degrees of tonicity than can be captured in descriptions of these degrees in propositions. Palpating a uterus for diagnostic purposes requires considerable practical knowledge. A nurse could only obtain this following experience of palpating several other uteruses previously.

This example lends very strong support to the view that practical knowledge resists specification in propositions. Recall, however, that it does not thereby follow that propositional knowledge is wholly irrelevant. Knowledge relating to the normal location of the uterus, the causes of differing degrees of tonicity and so on is plainly crucial here.

With regard to the question of how we are to determine whether or not a person possesses practical knowledge, Benner's view seems describable as follows. Recall our discussion of propositional knowledge (Chapter 2). We wondered there if, within the realm of practical knowledge, there could be a distinction analogous to that between knowledge and belief within the propositional realm (one between practical knowledge and practical 'belief' so to speak).

Within the propositional realm, beliefs can be distinguished in terms of grades of plausibility. The more plausible the belief, the closer it approximates to knowledge. Benner's 'five stages' in the transition from novice to expert might usefully be recruited here to articulate an analogous grading. Thus the novice and the expert differ in the extent to which their respective performances of a task will be successful. The expert's performances will be successful most (all?) of the time, and the novice's less so. And of course we have the grades between these levels – advanced beginner, and so on.

So within the realm of practical knowledge, 'knowledge' amounts to success in the performance of an activity A. And it can be supposed this performance has a certain smoothness of execution characteristic of experts and aspired to by novices. Thus it does seem possible to articulate an equivalent of the knowledge/belief distinction (more strictly, between more and less plausible beliefs) within the realm of practical knowledge. Having said this, what 'success' amounts to in the performance of a practical task in nursing is not unproblematic. This is a problem we return to shortly (in discussion of a charge of conservatism levelled at Benner's claims).

A further observation which Benner makes on the relationship between practical and theoretical knowledge is this. She claims that descriptive research (research set out in the form of written sentences), for example into expert nursing practice, can lead to the development of improved practice (for example, 1984, pp. 107, 166, 169). And at an earlier stage in nursing education, she is clear that it is beneficial to learn descriptive knowledge in biology and 'psycho-social sciences' (ibid., p. 184). Hence Benner does not endorse a position in which descriptive knowledge has no place within nursing practice or education.

An additional point of interest arises on the topic of practical knowledge as this is discussed within *FNE*. As mentioned earlier Benner includes within the realm of practical knowledge a wide range of phenomena. Most obviously these include the skilled performance of motor tasks such as giving injections, taking pulses and so on. Benner also includes types of activities such as inter-actions with patients at a different level, for example, bathing them, dressing them; and also adopting appropriate posture when dealing with them – for example if the patient is anxious and frightened. Still further, skills such as managing a ward all count as instances of practical knowledge for Benner.

This all seems very plausible. As with the 'palpating a uterus' example, it is reasonable to suppose that the kinds of skills and degrees of discernment necessary to manage a ward are such that they cannot exhaustively be speci-fied in lists of propositions.

However, it was suggested in Chapter 2 above that the distinction between practical and propositional knowledge is often cast in a number of *equivalent* ways (for example how/that; theoretical/practical; bodily/intellectual). But we have just seen that it is plausible to include knowledge of a skill such as managing a ward within the category of practical knowledge. Recall that the idea of *bodily* knowledge was explained in terms of bodily intentionality, in the representation 'within the body' of the relevant motor task. Examples of typing and playing a musical instrument were given to illustrate this. The idea of practical knowledge being explicated by reference to bodily intentionality sounds feasible when discussed in relation to some practical motor skill. But this sounds less plausible in relation to the kind of practical knowledge required to manage a ward. This seems more of a mental than a bodily task. If correct, this suggests that the category of practical knowledge is more general than that of bodily knowledge. So the propositional/practical distinc-tion is *not* cast equivalently when cast as a 'bodily/intellectual' distinction.[1]

With these clarifications now complete, we turn now to look more criti-cally at Benner's claims within *FNE*. We look specifically at two charges to which her views seem vulnerable: the first is the charge of conservatism, and the second is the charge of mysticism.

Further, against the complaint that the reconstrual of claims relating to knowledge as claims about belief are simply examples of excessive nit-picking, consideration of some of the claims made by Benner in relation to expert practice can help to show the value of using the term 'knowledge' sparingly and strictly.

Two criticisms of Benner's position within FNE

Conservatism

One complaint which has been levelled at Benner's work is that it fosters conservatism (Cash, 1995, p. 532; Paley, 1999). The justification for this charge is roughly as follows. Benner's position in relation to expertise is one in which one becomes an expert through manifestation of practice at a certain level. This is recognised and designated as such by relevant colleagues, and other expert practitioners. As we heard earlier, Benner also offers an explanation of how it is that the expert's practice differs from that of the novice. Once achieved, the status of expert remains provided one's performance does not significantly deteriorate.

Cash points out that these judgements relating to what constitutes expert practice necessarily presuppose some context within which they make sense. Thus recall the example given earlier in which we distinguished two nurses, one who proved extremely capable of defusing potentially violent episodes so they did not take place, and another who seemed to lack this capability. Suppose the first nurse acquires a reputation for expertise in this area of nursing, in dealing with aggressive patients; moreover, the nurse functions in a way which meets Benner's explanation of expertise: she possesses the relevant skills of intuitive judgement and action. Here it is evident that judgements concerning what amounts to expert practice are bound to presuppositions concerning just what a good nursing intervention is. Thus to describe this nurse's practice as expert because she is able to defuse aggressive situations presupposes it is considered good nursing so to defuse them. This point can be generalised to all instances of expert practice within nursing (and indeed beyond): judgements concerning what constitutes expertise are inseparable from judgements concerning what is considered good practice.

To see the concern which Cash has in relation to Benner's conception of expertise, the example just offered shows how defining expertise by reference to what is currently considered expert practice can merely serve to entrench current practices. For suppose it could be shown to be worse to defuse aggressive situations than to encourage them to be acted out. Perhaps on the ground that this, ultimately, has greater therapeutic value. It seems hard to see how such a change in practice can arise in Benner's position. The reason is that, as pointed out, it defines expert practice by reference to what is currently regarded as such.

More generally, recall that for Benner a characteristic of expert performance is seeing situations through a 'gestalt' or pattern. This amounts to the view that expert practice involves bringing to bear on situations a certain conceptual framework, one which has been developed over time, and which has been informed by the relevant past experiences of the practitioner. Within the context of Benner's discussion one can see how this can seem a positive aspect of the expert's role. But it can equally well be shown to be a negative feature of the expert's view. Benner's expert, it may be said, has a fixed, entrenched view; one not amenable to new developments and new ways of seeing situations. The reason is that it appears to be a virtue of Benner's expert that one sees situations through the conceptual lens one has found reliable in the past and through the application of which one has become known as possessing expertise.

One can see how this understanding of expertise leads to the charge of conservatism advanced by Cash, and of the difficulties of explaining changes in practice from within a Bennerian position. Benner's account appears simply to entrench current practice and impede revisions of it.

This is, in fact, reflected in some of the comments made by the people interviewed in *FNE*. One expert makes the following statement:

> When I say to a doctor, 'the patient is psychotic,' I don't always know how to legit-imise that statement. *But I am never wrong.* Because I know psychosis from the inside out. And I know it, and I trust it. I don't care if nothing else is happening, I still really know that (*FNE*, p. 32) (emphasis added).

Benner describes the person making this statement as 'an expert psychiatric nurse clinician' (1984, p. 32).

There are at least two concerns which may be prompted by this quote. A first one, illustrated in the sentence emphasised, is the confidence with which the nurse states that he or she is 'never wrong'. This is an extraordinarily strong claim. It also reinforces the worry to which Cash draws attention. How could a person who is convinced they are 'never wrong' (that is, in matters relating to their field of expertise) ever be persuaded to revise their practice? As far as they are concerned, since they are never wrong there is no need to revise it.

Second, the confidence with which this expert speaks is especially troubling since it is in the area of psychiatric diagnosis. The whole category of mental illness is itself highly controversial (see Szasz, 1972), and so too are the diag-nostic categories within it (see van Os et al., 1993). As I understand the current situation, traditional divisions between neuroses and psychoses are being subjected to serious critical scrutiny. The expert's claim to know psychosis 'from the inside out' is contentious at best. To know it from the inside suggests actual experience of psychotic illness, but there is no indication in the text that this is the claimed source of the expert's knowledge.

So this specific example of an expert's view of his or her own expertise, taken from *FNE*, seems to lend considerable support to the conservatism charge levelled at Benner's account by some critics. (Note that this criticism need not affect the point that conservatism can still be a virtue of theorising, as shown by Quine and Ullian.)

One way to explain what is going on in Benner's account of expertise is to point to a conflation of two different understandings of the 'status' of knowledge. In the first one, knowledge is viewed as unrevisable, as having the necessary connection with truth which we observed in our discussion of it. On this view of knowledge, it is almost impossible to obtain – due to the force of the sceptic's challenges – yet, if one did possess it one could exude the kind of confident certainty which is exuded by Benner's expert in the quote above.

On a second understanding of the concept of knowledge, one which is erroneous according to the view presented in Chapter 2, knowledge is in fact revisable. Thus on this view one could be said to know *p* at one time, and yet *p* turn out later to be false. I suspect that it is a view of knowledge of this kind with which, if pressed, Benner would admit to be presupposing. However, a view of knowledge of this kind entails a certain modesty in relation to what one claims to know. For according to it, at some future point one might be shown to be mistaken. But Benner's expert is not a modest one, but an immodest one; one who 'knows' they are never wrong.

So my suggestion here is this. We noted two models of knowledge, one which permits revisability and one which does not. The model which does not permit revisability due to the tightness of the relationship between knowledge and truth, fosters a kind of immodesty in relation to knowers: if they know they know, they know they cannot be wrong. This might then warrant the kind of certitude possessed by Benner's experts.

But it is not likely that Benner subscribes to this model of knowledge; it is more likely that she subscribes to the model in which knowledge is compatible with revisability (otherwise she would be much more cautious in her use of the term 'knowledge' in *FNE*). Subscription to this model entails a certain modesty, as shown above, since one might later be shown to be mistaken in what one 'knows'.

So the model of knowledge favoured by Benner does not warrant the degree of certitude manifested by her experts. One model of knowledge does warrant such a degree (that is, the model in which knowledge is not revisable) but Benner does not subscribe to this. The claim here is that the degree of certitude manifested by Benner's experts is, thus, not warranted. The fact that they manifest it can be explained by a confusion over just what it is that 'knowledge' means: something revisable, or something not.

Intuition and mysticism

The second area of criticism of Benner's work within *FNE* centres on her appeals to intuition. As reported earlier, the concept of intuition has proved a further source of controversy in her analysis of expertise. We noted that her text sustains at least two interpretations, one broadly mystical and one in which intuitive judgement is anchored in empirically available phenomena.

Quine and Ullian, interestingly, discuss exactly the kind of situation Benner exploits in her discussion. They describe situations in which 'though we are quite convinced that a belief is right, we can think of no reasons at all for holding it' (1978, p. 92); and they suggest that it is in situations of this kind that intuition is appealed to. This all concurs so far with Benner's discussion of expertise, in that, as we saw, experts make the same kind of claim as that referred to by Quine and Ullian.

Further, Quine and Ullian discuss the two interpretations of appeals to intuition set out above: one in which it is grounded in empirical data and one in which it is not. They observe, 'The appeal to intuition is explicit and most insistent... among devotees of doctrines that are short on reasoned support. Really there is no place for an explicit appeal to intuition. Where an intuition has anything at all to be said for it, it has something making no mention of intuition to be said for it...' (1978, p. 92). In other words, legitimate appeals to intuition are restricted to those where intuitive judgements stem from empirically available evidence, and since it is the presence of empirically available evidence which justifies the 'intuitive' judgement, and not the intuition, there is no need to appeal to intuition.

If this is considered unduly harsh, consider the consequences of allowing that intuitive judgements are legitimate even when not based upon any empirically discernible data. I might strike you on the grounds that my intuition 'told' me that you were about to attack me. Or, one might place a huge sum of money on a bet on a horse on the grounds that one 'intuitively knew' it would romp home in an easy victory. More seriously, it is surely a requirement of professional practice, in which practitioners are held to account for their actions, that they be able to offer explanations of their actions. This requirement seems a perfectly reasonable one, and it seems to demand at least the possibility of rational defence and explanation (for example as emerges from empirical studies of expert decision-making such as that referred to in English (1993)).

So, following Quine and Ullian and one way of reading of Benner, the notion of intuition can be seen to have some limited legitimacy, and not to be 'mystical', when it is grounded in empirically available data. Yet it should be said that the 'mystical' construal of intuition is still strongly associated with Benner's work. This is fostered in part by the availability of the two interpretations of intuition in *FNE*. And also by references to a 'sixth sense' (p. 23) in headings which accompany the 1987 paper by Benner and Tanner 'How expert nurses use intuition'. Even in this paper the two construals of intuition are available. As noted the paper is accompanied by references to a 'sixth sense', and intuition is defined as 'understanding without a rationale' (1987, p. 23).

Benner and Tanner explicitly deny that this is mystical in any way (1987, p. 23), but the definition they offer invites readers so inclined to the interpretation that intuition cannot be given a rationale. Yet, officially at least, Benner does seem committed to the view that it can be explained, and therefore, given a rationale. This need not entail that individual expert practitioners are capable of providing such explanations of their decision-making, but that as with the study on chess players, such a study would uncover relevant empirical data which can be shown to prompt their 'intuitive' judgements.

In these last two sections we have tried to bring to bear the philosophical work we undertook on the concept of knowledge onto the work of Carper and Benner. Considerable ground has been cleared. Hopefully, this will inform future discussion and assessment of these important contributions to philosophy of nursing.

In the final part of this chapter, we turn to the idea of nursing knowledge per se.

What is nursing knowledge?

Whatever nursing knowledge is, we have heard that knowledge itself is crucially related to truth. And, with reference to propositional knowledge for it to be true that S knows that *p*, then *p* must be true. Thus it is clear that knowing is importantly different from believing and opining: the latter two have no necessary connection to truth (it can be true that S believes or is of the opinion that *p* regardless of whether or not *p* is true).

With regard to practical knowledge, criteria for possession of this seem necessarily bound to the successful performance of the relevant task. This is the case whether or not such performances require propositional knowledge of the steps involved. Our criticism of Benner in the last section suggests that, as with propositional knowledge, experts in practical knowledge should maintain an attitude of modesty towards their performances such that the ends they aim at are essentially revisable. The most they can claim is that given *present conceptions* of ends, practical knowing of a certain kind K brings about ends E. It can be added that this claim should be extended to means also. Some means presently thought best to achieve ends E may be shown to be replaceable by some other set of means.

With reference to propositional knowledge, very strictly speaking this involves beliefs only, with varying degrees of plausibility. Therefore an attitude of modesty on the part of the 'knower' is required in this domain also.

Given these qualifications, let us conclude this chapter with a discussion of the whole idea of there being a specific body of knowledge which is 'nursing knowledge'.

Are disciplines defined by their objects of knowledge?

As noted earlier, at least part of the explanation of why it has seemed compelling to many nurse theorists to articulate a core of nursing knowledge is that spelling this out would help to distinguish nursing from other disciplines, especially the health-related professions – medicine, social work, physiotherapy and so on.

The enquiry into the nature of nursing knowledge is fuelled by a presumption such as that stated below by Parse; namely, that articulation of a corpus of knowledge which is unique to a discipline, is necessary for that discipline to have a clear and distinct identity:

> Every discipline has… a substantive core of knowledge that identifies it as a unique entity (1995, p. 51).

It follows from this, of course, that if nursing is to be a coherent, unified discipline there must be a 'substantive core' of the kind Parse envisages.

On the face of it, this does seem a plausible requirement. One of the ways in which disciplines seem distinguishable is by the identification of the objects with which the discipline is concerned, of which they seek knowledge and enquire into the natures of (Parse, 1987, p. 2).

For example, it is common to divide scientific enquiry into the physical sciences on the one hand, and the biological sciences on the other (see, for example, Asimov, 1984). Examples of physical sciences include, obviously, physics, astronomy, geology, meteorology and so on. Examples of biological sciences include, again obviously, biology, chemistry, psychology, anatomy and physiology and so on.

Roughly speaking, this highly general division rests upon a difference in the objects of which knowledge is sought: the physical sciences are concerned with inanimate ('non-living') matter, whereas the biological sciences are concerned with animate ('living') phenomena.

Having said this, it is worth bearing in mind the following point. All the objects in which the biological sciences are interested are ultimately composed of phenomena of interest to the physical sciences – sub-atomic particles; humans and other animals, for example, are ultimately composed of such particles. Yet it does not follow from this that the biological sciences are simply identical to the physical sciences and that, psychology, for example, is simply a branch of particle physics. Hence, it can be allowed that differing sciences can be interested in the same objects, even though these will be differently thought of in those sciences. For the particle physicist, a person is a collection of sub-atomic particles, but a psychologist, typically, would not view a person in such terms even though it can be allowed that persons are composed of such particles.

Parallel points could be made in relation to nursing: although the phenomena of concern to nurses are also ultimately composed of sub-atomic particles, it is not this level of categorisation of objects at which nursing focuses. So the identification of the categories with which a discipline is concerned appears to go some of the way towards identifying a discipline as distinct from other disciplines. To make this point as starkly as possible: nursing differs from astronomy in that the prime objects of concern to astronomers are planets and other heavenly bodies; but the prime concerns of nursing include persons (if they include planets at all, they do so only peripherally).

What, then, are the phenomena which are of prime interest to nursing? Persons, health, disease, and the environment are types of phenomena commonly cited as comprising the core phenomena of nursing (for example Nightingale, 1957; Parse, 1981; Fawcett, 1995, p. 7). But of course individually each one of these four is an important object of concern of some other discipline: psychologists are interested in persons, pathologists in disease, town planners in the environment. Moreover, public health doctors, it seems, can also claim to be interested in all four types of phenomena: persons, health, disease and the environment. Hence, the mere articulation of this specific realm of objects of concern is not sufficient to distinguish nursing from (at least) medicine.

So the attempt to define nursing by reference to its *objects* of key concern appears doomed to failure. The body of knowledge which comprises nursing knowledge, and which articulates the unique identity of nursing, is not to be found by the mere identification of the objects of knowledge of nursing. Perhaps, then, it is the nature of the relationship to these objects of concern which marks out the territory within which the domain of nursing knowledge is to be located and articulated.

Are disciplines defined by their ends?

Wartofsky (1992) has argued that 'human knowledge is teleological... It is acquired and used for the sake of some end' (p. 133). Trivially, it might be thought that the end for which knowledge is sought is the pursuit of truth; less trivially, for the sake of prestige and power. However we think the question of the most general ends of knowledge should be answered, Wartofsky proposes, with reference to medical knowledge, that:

> what distinguishes medical knowledge, what individuates it as medical, rather than as biological, historical or moral knowledge, is the distinctive ends that it serves (1992, p. 134).

So the ends of biology may, for example, be the control or domination of nature and biological knowledge is that which is deployed to that end. Consideration of the ends of medicine will help to determine what it is that distinguishes it from other disciplines. Hence, the proposal here is that disciplines can best be distinguished by reference to their ends. So we should not expect that a specification of the objects of medical knowledge will serve to individuate medicine. Rather, what is required is a specification of its ends.

Perhaps a similar strategy may prove of use in order to determine the distinctiveness of nursing knowledge.

Wartofsky suggests, plausibly, that although the ends of medicine have been subject to change, due to changes in social values, a constant concern can be detected with well-being and ill-being (1992, p. 135). These, in turn, he suggests are tied to human needs; that is to say, conceptions of what wellness and illness amount to will be determined by human needs. The claim that one is ill when one is not able to meet one's needs is, of course, a familiar one in nursing literature (Orem, 1971). And the proposal that disciplines can be individuated by reference to their ends, in contrast to their objects, opens up the promise of a strategy by which to distinguish medical and nursing knowledge. Even if they have the same objects, they may have different ends.

A major stumbling block with this proposal, however, is that it seems plausible that not only do medicine and nursing have the same objects, but they also share the same ends. They are each concerned to promote well-being and to relieve suffering and ill health. So even a focus on ends seems to fail to distinguish the medical and nursing enterprises.

Are the means by which nurses meet their ends distinctive?

A different strategy, however, is to focus on the *means* by which the respective enterprises seek to bring about their shared ends. Hence it may be possible to argue that the means by which nurses seek to bring about the shared ends of the nursing and medical enterprises differ importantly from the means employed by medical staff. It is fair to say that the concepts of care and cure have been recruited to try to effect this articulation (for example Liaschenko and Davis, 1991; Kuhse, 1997). But drawing the distinction itself has proved problematic (see Chapters 6 and 7), in part due to difficulties in specifying the content of the concept of care. Also many physicians quite properly reject the apparent implication of the claim that their main focus lies on cure. Of course, many medical personnel are not engaged in the business of curing patients (for example those working in terminal care, care of people with advanced dementia, and so on) and many maintain, justly, that they are as caring as any nurse in their practice.

So even though it seems that the means by which nurses seek to bring about the (shared) ends of the discipline is the most promising focus for an articulation of what nursing and nursing knowledge is, there remain problems in the attempt to articulate the distinctive means of nursing.

One interesting attempt to articulate the distinctive means by which nurses bring about the ends in nursing has been made by Malmsten (1999). Her contention is that 'basic care' is the most promising focus to identify the unique core of nursing knowledge referred to by Parse. Thus it may be argued that the knowledge involved in giving basic care constitutes the kind of core sought by Parse. By basic care Malmsten seems to mean the kinds of nursing activities which involve physical contact between the nurse and the patient. This may arise for example in washing, or shaving patients, in giving them pressure area care, and also in feeding them or helping them with feeding (Malmsten defines basic care as 'the kind of care that has to do with our bodily functions', 1999, p. 17). She asserts that it is this specific kind of caring activity which is distinctively the domain of the nurse. She proposes that other health care professionals – physicians, physiotherapists and so on – do not engage in this kind of basic care, at least to the extent to which nurses do.

Malmsten also points out that, by virtue of being unique to nursing, basic care underpins the autonomy of nursing (1999, p. 237). In other words, the distinctive role of nurses among other health care professionals can be articulated by reference to the performance of basic care.

Malmsten's attempt to set out what is unique to nursing is multifaceted and impressive. But it seems to me to suffer from a fairly fundamental flaw. This is as follows. Malmsten's is an attempt to unearth some activity or range of activities unique to nursing. Her claim is that this range of activities are those which lie within the category of basic care. But Malmsten's attempt seems another failure. It fails, first, for the reason that not all nurses are engaged in basic care. Thus, for example, a nurse working in a psychotherapy unit would be very unlikely to engage in basic care; nor would a nurse working in, say, the contexts of secure psychiatric nursing, or teaching social skills to people with mild intellectual disabilities. So not all nurses seem involved in the giving of basic care. But further, of course, some non-nurses are engaged in the giving of such care, for example, home carers – people caring for a chronically sick relative.

The claim that basic care is unique to nursing only succeeds if it is performed only by nurses, and by all nurses. As seen, neither of these claims is true. Therefore defining nursing by reference to basic care fails. So this attempt to unearth, at the level of means, the kind of knowledge base distinct to nursing also seems unsuccessful.

Moreover, as indicated in the discussion of Carper and Benner's work, practical knowledge is central to nursing. Yet this is held, by definition, to be unspecifiable. If this proves to be the case the prospects for describing the 'substantive core of knowledge' referred to by Parse in the quote given earlier seem dim. If Carper and Benner are correct nursing knowledge is such that it, in principle, resists description in propositional form.

It should be added that practical knowing seems equally intrinsic to medical practice, and yet its integrity as a discipline is not jeopardised by this. Thus a lesson which may be drawn from this discussion is that the integrity of a discipline need not require the specification of the 'substantive core' referred to in Parse's quotation.

Conclusion

Our discussion of knowledge and belief raises the problem of whether in the interests of precision to refrain wholly from use of the term 'know', especially in relation to empirical claims. Wherever we see the word 'know' should we substitute this with 'believe'? A term which signals that a claim is particularly well-established, or highly plausible, would be useful for purely pragmatic purposes. The employment of the term 'know' for such purposes seems reasonable. But as seen in our discussion of Benner, such claims to know must be accompanied by a degree of modesty with regard to what is being claimed as known. Recognising the essentially revisable nature of knowledge claims (especially empirical knowledge claims) can steer us away from vulnerability to charges of conservatism, and help keep (appropriately) at bay appeals to tradition and authority. This seems especially significant in nursing. As Rodgers (1991) indicates, appeals to tradition there are widespread. And equally, the recognition of the provisional nature of knowledge can help to counter the epistemic authority of the medical profession. For the revisability of knowledge applies in this domain also. Hence, as with all scientists, the claims of current medical orthodoxy are likely to be overturned at some future date.

The essential revisability of knowledge also maps onto the domain of practical knowing. As seen, the person with practical knowledge is distinguishable from the person who lacks it by reference to the success with which their acts achieve the ends sought in the relevant domain or practice. Since 'success' here is inseparable from a conception of ends aimed at, and since these may change (recall the 'violent episodes' example under the sub-heading *Two criticisms of Benner's position within FNE*) then revisability also applies here. This has the consequence that a degree of modesty is required of experts in relation to their expertise.

In general, then, we should note the revisability of knowledge claims within both propositional and practical realms. In the latter this applies at the level of ends and also at the level of means. Given this epistemological enquiry we can conclude that any credible account of nursing must respect our findings in these past two chapters. Having, thus, established a position regarding knowledge, we can now turn to the second main category of philosophy, ontology.

Our discussion of knowledge began with the observation that the body has been considered an obstacle to knowledge. This indicates how views regarding mind and body are related to conceptions of knowledge. As will be seen in our next chapter, views regarding the nature of nursing can be shown to be intrinsically bound to conceptions of what it is to be a person.

SUGGESTIONS FOR FURTHER READING

Texts on the nature of knowledge

The relevant chapters in Nagel, Grayling and Popkin and Stroll are all helpful here. But it is worth adding that the Quine and Ullian text referred to in the discussion within Chapters 2–3 presents a very clear, brief and accessible philosophical discussion of knowledge, and also philosophy of science.

D.W. Hamlyn's (1970) book *The Theory of Knowledge* is another, more difficult, although still accessible discussion of the topic. A more recent, comparable, introduction is R. Audi (1998) *Epistemology: A Contemporary Introduction to The Theory of Knowledge*, London: Routledge.

With regard to practical knowledge, Ryle's discussion in Chapter 2 of his *The Concept of Mind* (1949) Harmondsworth: Penguin, is extremely clear and accessible. And of course Benner's (1984) book should be seen as an important contribution to this area. Dunne (1993) provides a very thorough discussion of the idea of practical judgement in the most general sense, that is, as combining both practical and propositional knowledge.

4 Nursing the person (i): ontology

This chapter and the next centre on the concept of a person.[1] In the present chapter we attempt to describe an adequate ontological account of persons. The purpose of this is to place subsequent discussion of persons on a secure ontological footing. This will require us (in the second part) to consider the mind–body problem and four main responses to it.

Introduction

As already noted, commentators such as Benner and Wrubel, and Parse expressly favour a Merleau-Pontian ontology of the person. Typically, their promotion of this stems from rejection of Cartesian dualism and a fairly crude reductionist view of persons (in which it is held that persons are 'nothing but' biological organisms, say). It will be suggested here that the move to embrace a Merleau-Pontian account is premature. Given the 'virtues' described by Quine and Ullian (Chapter 2 above) a more modest position is recommended. The more modest line is one which allows that mental properties (thoughts, feelings and so on) are *dependent upon* physical ones (for example brain states), but which denies they are *reducible to* brain states (that is, denies that they are 'nothing but' brain states). As will be seen, this position avoids the problems which beset Cartesian dualism, and the crude reductionist position but does not require the wholesale revision of thought about the mind and body called for by the Merleau-Pontian position.

Having established a (relatively) secure ontological basis for an account of persons, we turn in the next chapter to develop a narrative account of personal identity. As will be seen, this has particular cogence for nursing, and health care work more generally.

According to Benner and Wrubel, 'theories of nursing practice, ..., are all based on assumptions about what it is to be a person' (1989, p. 28). One obvious way in which Benner and Wrubel's claim is true is this. Interventions which aim at giving persons nutrition, or making them comfortable all presuppose persons are the kinds of things which benefit from being given nutrition, and which prefer to be comfortable.

But of course Benner and Wrubel are getting at a deeper point than this. Their claim is that differences in philosophical presuppositions regarding what persons are can be discerned, and these differences can be shown to generate differing conceptions of nursing.

To see this consider a concept fundamental to nursing, that of health. According to one theory of health – a biostatistical theory – health consists simply in the absence of disease. And disease is defined in terms of the proper function of a human considered as a biological organism. Hence, any physical lesion which impugns the function of a bodily system constitutes a disease (for example a kidney tumour or a pathogenic micro-organism). One is healthy on such a view when one is 'disease free'. (See Greaves, 1996 for a critical account of this theory.)

A clear implication of this view of health is that the question of whether or not a person is healthy can be determined simply by examination of that person; that is, a person considered as nothing more than a biological organism. There is no need to engage with the person, so to speak. Physical examination will reveal whether or not they are healthy. This is the case regardless of the person's own view of the matter. Moreover, it seems to follow from the theory that biological equivalence entails 'health' equivalence. In other words, if two persons have the same biological state, whether of disease or of the absence of disease, their health status must be the same too. It seems to follow further, that the nursing care they require will also be the same. For if two cases are equivalent, what could be the rationale for treating them differently on this theory?

This account of health views humans as essentially biological organisms. And such a view requires that an identifiable physical cause – a disease – is present for it to be the case that a person is legitimately describable as ill.

According to a second view of health, concepts such as well-being and quality of life are typically appealed to. And in this view, sometimes described as a holistic view, much more emphasis is given to the subjective feelings, values and aspirations of persons. (Again, see Greaves, 1996.) From the perspective of this second account, health consists in much more than simply the absence of disease. And, typically, this account of health is proposed to derive from an opposition to what is regarded as the crude reductionism of the first account.

This holistic account of health also derives from a view of persons such that they are more than simply biological systems. So on this view, in opposition to the biostatistical view, the question of whether or not a person is healthy cannot be determined simply by physical examination of that person, considered as a biological organism. On this view, it seems, engagement with the person at some other level is required. Similarly, on the holistic view, equivalence in health status cannot be inferred from biological equivalence. And further, biological equivalence does not entail equivalence in the planned nursing care of persons. (See Chapter 5 where we distinguish biological from narratival understanding.)

More positively, the holistic view of what health amounts to derives from a particular, non-reductionist account of what it is to be a person. According to the account, persons are defined partly by their values and aspirations or goals. When their capacity to pursue these goals is compromised (for example by a lesion within the body), and when this is felt by the person concerned, this is considered indicative of ill-health.

It is worth stressing again an important difference in the two views of health just described. In the first view, the question of whether or not a person is genuinely ill can be answered simply by examining that person. But in the holistic view it is necessary, at least, to take into account what the person's own view of the matter is. In the holistic account, the question of a person's health/illness is not detachable from that person's own view of the matter.

Hence the two views of what it is to be a person, the reductionist and non-reductionist, can be shown to foster differing views of what health consists in, and differing views on how to determine whether or not a person is ill. The first view requires no input from the person concerned. The second view appears to require such input.

To relate these reflections more explicitly to nursing, consider an 'Oremesque' conception of persons as essentially needs-bearers, where for the sake of simplicity we construe needs as physical needs. Needs generate 'self-care requisites' such as those for water, food and air. In states of ill health persons become unable to meet these and so develop self-care deficits.

Ill health, in this view, disrupts a person's capacity to meet their own needs, and thus to care for themselves. Hence, kidney disease would impinge upon the need for proper metabolism of fluid. This conception of persons and of illness then generates a view of nursing such that nurses must endeavour to meet those needs of patients that they are not themselves capable of meeting, due to their illness.

Note that no reference to the patient's own view on the significance of these deficits occurs in this account. But it seems plain that at the biological level two patients might have the same problem, say a broken ankle, but that the significance of this would be greater for one patient than for another – for example if the patient is a professional dancer. So if persons, and thereby patients, are viewed in exclusively biological terms, from a nursing viewpoint, two patients with the same biological problems (self-care deficits) present the same nursing problems and require the same types of nursing interventions. But the 'dancer' example suggests that what constitutes a good nursing intervention requires more than mere consideration of patients in biological terms.

Thus in support of Benner and Wrubel's observation, we see how at a very basic level, conceptions of persons lead to conceptions of nursing.

Some views of the person in nursing

Having considered some examples in support of Benner and Wrubel's claim, consider now some differing conceptions of the person to be found within nursing literature.

The first is a view ascribed to Henderson by McKenna. He suggests Henderson views persons as 'Biological human beings with inseparable mind and body...' (1997, p. 243; Henderson, 1966, see p. 11). This raises a puzzle. Since 'biological' normally indicates something physical, it seems to follow that if persons are biological, and have minds, then minds are wholly physical, and so are persons too. So this *appears* to be a reductionist view. One in which persons are biological entities and in which mind and body can be cast in biological terms.

A second view is put forward by Roy. For her, persons are conceived of as 'bio-psycho-social' beings (Roy, 1980, p. 180). Thus, in this, a person is a composite of broadly mental and physical items.

A third view is put forward by Watson. She espouses a position according to which mind and body are *separable*: 'A person's body is confined in space and time, but the mind and soul are not confined to the physical universe' (Watson, 1988, p. 50). And 'The spirit, inner self, or soul (geist) of a person exists in and for itself' (ibid.). (See also Holden, 1991.) So here the person is identified with the non-physical component, with the soul or spirit. Moreover, it is held that the person can survive without the physical component.

A fourth view is that with which Benner and Wrubel, and Parse, express sympathy. It is a view in which body and mind are held to be inseparably intertwined, to form one type of substance (Merleau-Ponty, 1962, 1968). Hence, it is not a view like that ascribed to Henderson or Roy. Nor is it a view like that of Watson's since that supposes mind to be categorically distinct from body.

So which of these views is correct? Henderson's (apparently) reductionist view, Roy's composite view, Watson's view of persons as souls, or Benner and Wrubel's Merleau-Pontian view? We will shortly go through four main positions in relation to this issue, but prior to this let us rehearse very briefly a 'commonsense' view. In this, I suspect, it would be held that persons are composed of mental and physical 'parts', so to speak (as comprising a mind and a body). And such a view seems reflected within health provision. Services are divided into those concerned with general, bodily, medicine, and those concerned with mental health. A division is supposed between mind and body: one set of services directed primarily at the body and the other primarily at the mind. And of course this is represented in nurse training, with there being separate training and qualifications for general and for psychiatric nurses.

Relatedly, it is common to distinguish physical from intellectual disabilities – sensory disabilities could presumably fit into either category.

So an important distinction seems presupposed in the way we think about health services, and this seems grounded in a view of the person such that persons are composites of a mind and a body. Yet, as we have seen, a range of views of the person are represented in nursing literature, at least one of which conflicts with the intuitive, commonsense line.

Consideration of what it is to be a person rapidly brings us to face the mind–body problem. The reason is that it simply does seem very plausible to consider persons to have minds and bodies. This then raises the question of what the relationship could be between these components, and it is this which generates the cluster of questions which comprise the mind–body problem. It is to this topic that we now turn.

After summarising the nature of the problem, four possible solutions to it are considered. As will be seen, none is without problems.

What's the problem?

In discussion of the problem it will be helpful to note a logical 'rule' which is tacitly presupposed in the following discussion. Crudely, the rule describes a constraint on all identity claims; that is, on claims in which it is said of two things that they are the same thing; in the present case, the two things are mind and body. According to the rule, if two things are identical, then they must have all their properties in common.

Three problems which form part of the mind–body problem are as follows. Note that the problems presume the logical rule just described to the effect that if two things really are the same, then they must have the same properties. The problems point to cases where it seems the mind has properties which physical things such as brains and bodies lack, or vice versa, and hence, given the logical rule just noted, they cannot be the same.

1. We each seem to have open to us a way of thinking about our own thoughts which, in principle, is not accessible to anyone else. Physical phenomena are accessible to all suitably equipped observers. But our own mental states are not accessible in the same way in which our physical states are. Therefore, our minds cannot be physical and cannot be identical with our brains or bodies – that is, since the logical rule described is plainly violated.

2. When one feel pains and other sensations, there is a distinctive way this feels. Yet, when brain states – neural connections and so on – are scrutinised, this 'felt' aspect is elusive, is not seen. Therefore, these sensations cannot be mere physical states.

3. The relations between one's thoughts are characterised in terms of their rationality. Hence, one's actions are explained by positing reasons for them. Such reasons for action are typically beliefs and desires. However, the relations between physical events are explained causally, in terms of the laws of nature. The behaviour of physical things is determined by natural laws; the behaviour/actions of persons is determined by their criteria of rationality. Therefore, mental states cannot simply be physical states.

These are the kinds of puzzles which generate a cluster of problems described as the mind–body problem.

Problems 1–3 suggest that the mind is not *identical* to the brain or body. Yet it is plain that they are related in some fundamental way. For it seems clear that there is mind–body causation, as in my deciding to move my arm; and also that there is body–mind causation, as when a burnt finger causes a sensation of pain. So it is very likely that the mind and the body are related, but specifying the nature of this relationship has proved a further element of the mind–body problem. It is possible to identify four main options.

Four accounts of the person

Persons as biological organisms

A first view is one in which persons are conceived of as essentially biological organisms. On this view, persons do not have non-physical minds or souls or spirits. For proponents of this view, mental phenomena such as thoughts and feelings are (identical to) simply physical states, typically brain states. This view seems reasonably described as a reductionist view. For according to it, mental phenomena (our thoughts, feelings, perceptions) are nothing more than physical phenomena such as chemical reactions in the brain. More technically, on this view of the person it is held that types of mental states are identical with types of brain states. Hence it is sometimes termed a 'type identity thesis' (see for example Armstrong, 1968; Wilson, 1979).

Thus on this view, all diseases are physical; as are all illnesses (that is, since all mental 'experiences' are physical ones). All treatment will presumably be aimed at changing some physical states of the person, since these will constitute the illness of the person.[2]

A view of the person of this kind is often attributed to a medical model or biomedical view of the person, for example:

> According to the medical model, a person is a complex set of anatomical parts (the lungs, liver, heart, and so on) and physiological systems (the respiratory system, the cardiovascular system, and so on) (Aggleton and Chalmers, 1986, p. 12; also Greaves, 1996).

Here the person is a wholly physical thing, a biological organism composed of biological subsystems. Disease is understood as physical – for example as a deviation in biological function (see Boorse, 1975) – and feelings of illness are simply reducible to physical states.

So following the intuition that persons are a composite of mind and body led us to consider just what the relations are between these two composite parts. According to the view of the person attributed to a medical model, the 'mind part' is simply reducible to the 'body part' – standardly the brain: all descriptions of the mind part can be redescribed fully in physical terms.

Thus, consider pain as an example of a type of mental state; and take *N*-states as a (fictional) example of a type of brain state. According to the view of mental–physical relations we are currently considering (mind-brain identity theory) pain is identical with *N*-states. So any particular pain state will be identical with an *N*-state.

Hence, in principle it will be possible to detect when a person is in pain by observing, with the relevant neurological scanner or sophisticated EEG, when a person's *N*-states are active, or are 'firing'. On this view, it is supposed that all other types of mental states can be conceived of along these same lines. It is, thus, worth emphasising that this kind of identity thesis is reductionist in that it holds mental phenomena to be identical to physical phenomena: that the mind simply *is* the brain or body.

This idea has proved highly seductive. For it seems supported by much empirical evidence concerning neurological and cognitive function, for example with reference to degenerative diseases such as dementia and Parkinsonism. Also, areas of the brain have been identified as having a specific responsibility for certain functions, for example the visual processing areas, and auditory processing areas (see, for example, Gross, 1987 pp. 391–2 on the localisation of brain function).

Some criticisms

However, certain standard objections have been levelled at the kind of position in which mental states are claimed to be reducible to brain states. First, it should be said that the neurophysiological data referred to above regarding diseases such as Parkinsonism and so on, do not in fact show that mental states simply *are* brain states. All they suggest is that the proper functioning of certain types of brain states appears to be necessary for certain mental functions. This falls far short of showing that those mental states are identical to those brain states. Imagine reasoning thus: oxygen is necessary for human life, therefore oxygen is identical with human life. This plainly does not follow. Something can be a necessary condition of a thing and not be identical with that thing. Another example: my father is a necessary condition of my existence, yet we are not the same person!

A second objection, directed at the claim that mental states are identical to brain states, stems from the possibility of variable realisation. Identity, it is claimed, is a relation of necessity; the properties which serve to identify a thing are essential to it, not merely contingent (that is, they are the properties a thing must possess in order to be that same thing). Given this understanding of the identity relation it is then pointed out that the relationship between any type of mental state and any type of brain state is likely to be contingent and not necessary. For example, suppose we come across a person who displays all the usual kinds of pain behaviours but who lacks N-states. Surely, it would not be denied that he was experiencing pain. Similarly, suppose a person's EEG revealed that his N-states were firing in the way in which they do when a person is in pain, yet the person denies he is in pain – he appears totally relaxed. Again, it is likely that the first-person reports of pain will trump the empirical data. This should not be surprising given that it seems part of the very meaning of 'pain' that it is something felt, experienced (Kripke, 1972).

Third, brain states themselves seem at least potentially open to view. We can envisage removing parts of the skull of a person in order to examine their brain. Hence brain states are at least potentially accessible to, can be viewed from, the third person perspective. But this seems not to be true of mental states. Pain is a good example of this. The experience of pain is private. For example I might be in pain, but not want to display this. But further, there seems a kind of access which I have to my pain states which is unique to me. No one can experience my pain in the way in which I myself do. Such states are accessible from the first-person perspective in a way which differs fundamentally to their accessibility from the third person perspective.

All this poses difficulties for the view that pain states are identical to brain states. For if, as our logical rule dictates, two phenomena are identical, whatever is true of one, should be true of the other. So if pain states are brain states, they should share all characteristics. Yet they seem not to. Pain states have a private, first-person accessibility which is crucial to their very nature – that is, it is what makes them what they are – and yet which is lacked by brain states. This counts further against the reductionist view.

A third, perhaps deeper, objection runs as follows. This concerns mental states such as beliefs that water is wet, or that Swansea is west of Cardiff, and so on – so-called intentional states. Recall that the type identity theorist must maintain that these too are identical to types of brain states. However, it is argued that the identities of such intentional states derive from the relations which their bearers (persons) have to their environment. Hence, if the environment differed, then their intentional states would differ too. This suggests that the identities of intentional states are determined in part by how things are outside the head/brain of the thinker. Given this, the nature of intentional states cannot be determined wholly by the relevant type of brain state; and this latter is required for it to be the case that intentional states, as a type of mental state, are identical with a type of brain state.[3]

Fiser (1986) makes a point of this kind concerning pain. Her claim is that the experience of pain is not independent of factors outside the brain of the person, namely the cultural context and linguistic discriminations present in the sufferer's linguistic community. Thus two people may be identical physically (that is, be undergoing the same types of brain states) yet one suffer intense pain, and another suffer less intense pain. Fiser's point is that responses to pain, and even the experience of pain itself cannot be severed from the cultural context of the person (also Cassell, 1991). Again this tells against the 'identity' view for in this, if two humans are physically identical they should be psychologically identical. Yet it seems we can envisage situations in which the nature of the mental states experienced by a person differ, due to cultural and other environmental factors, yet where his brain states are the same. It seems to follow that mental states cannot be identical with brain states.

In summary, the phenomena which are central to healthcare work – pain, suffering, well-being, and meaning (that is, the significance patients attribute to their symptoms and to their experiences) – have a personal, subjective, aspect to them which is crucial to their nature. Yet this aspect is such that it cannot be accommodated within the view which reduces mental states to mere physical states. For this requires the 'objectifying' of mental states, and one cannot do this without distorting their nature.

Given all these difficulties, there seem good reasons not to accept a view of persons such that they are merely physical, biological organisms. We now move on to consider a second view.

Persons are composed of mental and physical properties, but the former are not reducible to the latter: a dependence view

Consider now a position which attempts to respect the empirically close relations between mental and physical states, but to avoid the difficulties which beset the reductive theory just considered. This view is one in which it held that mental properties are *dependent upon* physical ones, but denies that mental properties are reducible to (simply *are*) physical ones. So on such a position it can be allowed that, say, a functioning nervous system is necessary for a person to have thoughts and feelings and hence that mental states are dependent upon brain states. But in this view it would be denied that mental states simply are brain states. Thus the kinds of chemical changes which take place in the nervous system may be necessary for thoughts and feelings, but thoughts and feelings are 'more than' simply chemical changes in the nervous system.

(Such a view is variously described as anomalous monism, non-reductive monism, or *token identity theory*. As we have heard, it is a view which acknowledges the dependence of mental properties (thinking, feeling and so on) upon physical ones, but rejects the view that mental properties are *reducible* to physical ones.)

This 'dependence' position has the merit of anchoring mental states within the physical world, and also, at the same time, of allowing the special nature of them – for example, their first-person accessibility, their non-reducibility to physical states and so on. So the position appears to respect what seem to be these two key conditions of an ideal theory.

On the downside, as McGinn (1982, p. 29) points out, the position is weak in the sense that it provides no account of the relations between mental and physical properties – other than bare dependence. McGinn describes the difficulty this way:

> Thus token-identity [the dependence view] on its own is compatible with the following possibility: that two creatures could have precisely the same physical properties, down to the microstructure of their brains, and yet have no mental properties in common... (ibid., p. 29).

He points out that this is unsatisfactory. For, we tend to suppose that if two things are alike physically, then they will be alike mentally. McGinn suggests that there are good reasons for such a supposition. For example, consider the possibility, allowed by our 'dependence view' (token identity theory) as described so far, that two people's thoughts differed yet they were physically identical. Since their thoughts differ, so will their behaviours, it is reasonable to suppose (for example if you desire water and I desire juice our thoughts will differ and so will our actions: you will walk to the water-dispenser and I will go to the juice-dispenser). But if the subjects are physically identical, their behaviours must presumably also be identical. So there seems a limit to the extent to which two persons could be identical physically and yet differ mentally. The dependence view, as described so far, seems incapable of accommodating this.

One response to the difficulty is to 'tighten up' the relations between mental and physical properties in some way. The relationship of supervenience has been posited to play this role. According to it: 'mental properties cannot vary while physical properties are kept constant' (McGinn, 1982, p. 29). So on this view any change in mental properties results from a change in physical properties. Moreover, it implies that psychological identity is determined by physical identity: that is, that 'sameness of physical attributes implies sameness of mental attributes' (ibid., p. 30) – although not vice versa.

While this is a tightening up of the relations between the two types of properties, it still leaves much unexplained and there have been many discussions and criticisms of the dependency view and its appeal to supervenience (see Macdonald and Macdonald, 1995). One key difficulty lies in explaining mind-to-body causation from within the approach (that is, the kind of causal sequence that is thought to occur when, say, one decides to move a part of one's body). In such causal sequences it appears as though the mind causes the bodily movements which result from a decision to move. However, it is problematic to reconcile this conception of mind-to-body causation with supervenience (see, for example, Kim, 1995). For in this type of causal sequence a mental change seems to precede a physical change and such a possibility appears ruled out by the supervenience relation; in this, the direction of determination is physical to mental. Of course body-to-mind causation is not problematic within this position since here a physical change results in a mental change, and this generates no difficulties with the requirements of the supervenience relation.

So this position, also, is not without difficulties it seems. It is not necessary for our purposes to pursue these difficulties. We have heard a bare description of the position and we can move on having noted a point of controversy which besets the position.

Persons are essentially minds or souls

The third position to be mentioned here holds that mind and body are essentially independent. Thus although a person is composed of a mind and a body, it is the survival of the mind which is both a necessary condition of the survival of the person, and a sufficient condition.

As noted earlier, this is a view championed within nursing literature by Watson (1988) and also Holden (1991). It is probably the French philosopher Descartes (1596–1650) who is the most famous traditional proponent of a view such as this. According to him, mind and body are essentially distinct. His claim is that there are only two kinds of substance: mind and material substance. The distinguishing, unique, feature of mind is its capacity to think, and the distinguishing, unique, feature of matter is its being spatial, it occupies space. Hence mind and body must be different since the former is a kind of non-spatial 'spirit' or soul-stuff, whereas the latter is non-thinking, space-occupying stuff.

It does not matter for our purposes how Descartes arrived at this view, but it has proved tremendously influential (recall the point made earlier concerning the structure of health service provision). And it is generally claimed to generate a view of medical practice according to which the primary focus of such practice is patients' bodies, and not patients themselves, a view which has come under serious criticism in recent years (Benner and Wrubel, 1989; Cassell, 1991).

For obvious reasons, Descartes' position is termed Cartesian dualism. In support of it it should be said that parts of it accord with many commonsense views about the mind, especially religious views. In these, for example, it is often held that the soul inhabits the body and leaves it at the point of death. Also, commonsense views of the mind frequently hold that the mind can on occasion 'insulate' itself against the body, for example, in periods of extreme suffering due to illness, or torture, or in meditative states and so on. Also, as noted, it is a position which appears to be supported by notable figures such as Watson (1988) and Holden (1991).

It should be said, however, that there are insuperable problems with this kind of Cartesian view. The most obvious one, as Descartes recognised ('Sixth

Meditation', 1954, p. 117), derives from the difficulty of explaining how mind and body can possibly interact. How can non-spatial mind causally effect spatial matter? Also, compared to views which bind the mind to the brain or the body, dualism seems a highly mysterious view. The former views can show how neural degeneration or development correlate with levels of cognitive function. But dualism renders this a complete mystery. For if the mind can survive in the absence of the body, why should the absence of specific parts of the brain have the kinds of catastrophic consequences to the mind which arise in serious brain injury and disease (for example dementia).

In short, dualism is constitutionally incapable of generating an explanation of a fundamental feature of our experience – that is, mind–body interaction – and this is a serious shortcoming.

Also, although it is true of Watson that she endorses a very strong version of this position, Holden adopts it for largely negative reasons. Reasonably enough, she seeks a position within philosophy of mind which does not reduce the mental domain to the merely physical. Thus phenomena such as pain, suffering and meaning she supposes, cannot simply be physical. And she suggests that attention to this domain is characteristic of the art of nursing. Moreover, in order to preserve a role for the science of nursing, she wishes to retain a view in which the mental domain is not severed from the physical. In spite of this, she advocates Cartesian dualism, a position in which the separability of the mental and physical domains is a key tenet.

The kind of 'dependence' view described in this section, is one which a theorist such as Holden should find attractive. It is non-reductive and so avoids the kind of view of the relationship between the mental and physical domains she is opposed to. And yet it does not sever completely the two domains; the mental is anchored in the physical. Holden can thus subscribe to a position in which the artistic and scientific dimensions of nursing are retained without endorsing the excesses of Cartesian dualism.

Persons are 'body subjects' in which mind and body are inseparably 'intertwined'

As noted, this is a thesis developed by Merleau-Ponty (1962, 1968) and is appealed to by Benner and Wrubel (1989, for example, p. 21) and Parse (1981, for example, p. 7; 1998).

Merleau-Ponty's position is notoriously difficult to set out. This is partly due to the fact that a dualism between the mental and physical is inherent in our language. Even the term 'intertwined' does not accurately describe Merleau-Ponty's position for it still implies an intertwining of two different types of stuff/properties. And for him, mental and physical properties are inseparable, and are mutually constitutive: each is infused with the other such that they comprise a seamless whole.

Further, according to Merleau-Ponty, the person is simply the body; more technically, his view is one according to which the body is a subject and not a mere object. This is in contrast with the previous three views. In these it seems that the person (that is, that which makes us the individual we are) lies in either the soul or brain. Thus the body is a mere instrument of the person (that is, the person being the brain or soul). Hence, on views 1–3 the body (excluding the brain) seems to be an object, and only contingently related to the person. By contrast, in Merleau-Ponty's view the whole of the body and the person comprise the same entity: a subject, not an object; and the person is not an entity composed of two separately identifiable components, one mental, one physical.

In spite of its obscurity, here are three types of considerations which may lend some support to this position.

Merleau-Ponty suggests that there is an 'organic relationship between subject and world' (1962, p. 152) and that there are 'intentional threads' (ibid., p. 136) which run from the body to objects. These threads partly constitute both the subject and the objects within the situation. The subject is, so to speak, moulded into the world; the character of the mould is not determined solely by the subject, but also by the nature of the world – hence, Merleau-Ponty's reference to an 'organic relationship... ' (ibid., p. 152).

One, perhaps overly simplistic, example of this is to note the form which our immediate environment takes. Cups are designed to be grasped, desks to be sat at, keyboards to be typed on and so on.

Also, the proposal that mind and body are inseparably intertwined seems extremely plausible. As seen above (Chapter 2), philosophers other than Merleau-Ponty have pointed to the phenomenon of bodily intentionality, such that in performing certain habitual activities it seems as though a kind of 'bodily knowledge' is being recruited.

Further, the view of the self as a unitary self (Hall, 1983, p. 345) again seems a plausible one. There does seem a fairly clear sense in which vision, for example, is not detachable from tactile and auditory senses. And it is plausible that the characteristic unity of our experience derives from overlapping relations between sensory and motor skills, rather than that of a simultaneous coordination of wholly distinct sensory and motor modules (for example as is supposed in a modular conception of mind (Fodor, 1983)).

Finally, Merleau-Ponty's account of the nature of the relationship between the person and the world also seems to match our usual understanding of that relationship. For example, to refer again to skilled behaviours, there is a sense in which a musician, say, becomes part of the instrument, or where, in cricket, the bat becomes part of the batsman. These examples indicate that the nature of a person's interaction with the world is typically of this char-acter. When one is walking, or cycling or picking up an object, speaking, seeing, and so on, one's actions are normally unreflective and yet exhibit a smoothness and ease which is of the same degree as the expertise shown by, for example, the musician in a different setting.

Also with reference to the experience of illness and of disability, Merleau-Ponty's position helps us to appreciate how these can be viewed as threatening the whole integrity of the person. For the threat to the body posed by illness and disability is a threat to oneself, to the person that one is. Hence the deep significance of some kinds of illness is easier to grasp given a Merleau-Pontian understanding of the person.

Some concluding remarks are called for on this brief account of Merleau-Ponty's position. It needs to be borne in mind that his philosophical stand-point is one of phenomenology. He describes his own project as one within the phenomenological movement (1962, preface). The key aim of this approach to philosophy is to describe experience as it really is – not to explain or analyse it (ibid., p. viii). Importantly, it is held that attempts to explain such phenomena necessarily distort them, for example compress them into categories artificially, make distinctions which are not reflected in reality. So scientific and philosophical descriptions impede true accounts of experience; only the phenomenologist recognises this and attempts to resolve it.

The same complaint is voiced against ordinary 'commonsense' thought. Merleau-Ponty urges us to place 'in abeyance the assertions arising out of the natural attitude [that is, our ordinary commonsense view of the world]' (ibid., p. vii); and to 're-achieve a direct and primitive contact with the world' (ibid.).

So with regard to Merleau-Ponty's position, phenomenology is a philo-sophical programme the aim of which is to describe experience as it actually is untainted by the lens of any theory – scientific, philosophical or common-sense. When this is done, when we reflect upon our experience we do not encounter a self separable from the world, but one which is inextricably bound to the world; similarly, we do not encounter a self which is divided into a separable soul and body, but a unified self. Philosophical enquiry misleadingly separates these elements of our experience which, in fact, are inseparable: mind, body and world.

Three fairly obvious objections to this line run as follows: first, surely all descriptions of experience involve some classification and categorisation of it. Hence, even phenomenological description may be distorting.

Second, what follows from the fact that we describe our experience as involving a unified self – that is, a self which is itself a unity and which is inseparably bound up with its environment? Surely, it may be objected, such descriptions may be false.

Third, against the Merleau-Pontian view, surely in some conditions our phenomenological experience suggests that we *are* distinct from our bodies. For example, in serious illness or disability it may be felt that the body is simply an obstacle to the person; its disability prevents the person pursuing the projects which they wish to pursue. (See for example Gadow, 1982 and her comments on 'the object body', p. 88.) A fascinating example of this is provided by J.D. Bauby (1997) in his book *The Diving Bell and the Butterfly*. The author suffers from so-called 'locked in syndrome'; in this his body remains paralysed, save for one eyelid, but his mind remains active. Phenomenologically, it seems here that the person's mind is intact while his body is clearly not. Yet such a dualist description must be incorrect according to the Merleau-Pontian line.

There are two responses which may be made to these objections. First, as Priest indicates (1998, p. 69), the phenomenologist can respond by suggesting that his project is to provide a description of experience which is *as free as possible* from distorting categories. Hence, the force of the objection can be acknowledged and efforts made to minimise it.

In response to the second objection, it can reasonably be claimed that the phenomenologist's task is to describe experience as it is. The question of its being mistaken is thus avoided. In other words, to what could an accurate phenomenological description be compared? It can only be compared to actual experience. The further question of theorising this experience is one which the phenomenologist rejects. That is where scientific and philosophical accounts of experience have gone wrong; they suppose their analyses provide a 'truer' account of experience. but this is a mistake in the eyes of the phenomenologist.

The third objection will, presumably, be countered by an argument to the effect that an *adequate* phenomenological analysis of (say) Bauby's experiences will reveal them to possess an inescapably bodily element.

With specific reference to attempts to employ Merleau-Ponty's position within nursing, Benner and Wrubel spend as much time as anyone explaining their reasons for adopting it. These may be summarised roughly as follows.

The first is that persons cannot be understood if regarded as objects (1989, p. 41). This is due to the centrality of concepts such as suffering, meaning and pain which appear to have an important subjective, private, aspect to them. Since the Merleau-Pontian view regards persons as subjects, the requirement not to regard humans as objects is met.

Second, nursing crucially involves much knowing how, for example in the performance of nursing skills. This appears to point to the significance of 'embodied intelligence' (ibid., p. 42). Within a Cartesian dualist position this expression sounds straightforwardly contradictory. For the concept of intelligence is mental and the body is by definition non-mental. The Merleau-Pontian line, however, accommodates such an idea extremely well. As we noted above, in this the body is not a mere object incapable of knowledge, but is a body-subject.

Third, more negatively, the Cartesian picture implies a certain model of the cognitive processes of persons. Thus perception is conceived of as information processing derived from representations of the outside world provided by the senses. And the person is to be understood:

as an agent who engages in rational calculation to determine what goals to set and how to attain them, and the journey through the life course is conducted on the basis of a cost-benefit analysis (1989, p. 51).

So here the person is an agent who engages in such calculations on the basis of information processed. The Merleau-Pontian line, by contrast, does not entail such a view of persons. In this view, one cannot separate the person from the context. Within the Merleau-Pontian position:

> The person is a creature of significance, constituted by relationships, meanings, and memberships, in short, a creature of culture (1989, p. 52).

Thus within the Cartesian picture a person can be defined without reference to their cultural context, but not so in the Merleau-Pontian view.

Let us briefly reconsider these three sets of considerations which Benner and Wrubel invoke to motivate the adoption of a Merleau-Pontian rather than some other position within philosophy of mind. As will be seen, my suggestion will be that the position we described as the 'dependence view' (alternatively, token identity theory) can be shown to have the merits which Benner and Wrubel find only in the Merleau-Pontian view.

First, regarding the importance of not viewing persons as objects. The strongly reductionist mind-brain identity theory described first above seems to have such an implication. In principle, on that position, all mental phenomena will be rendered accessible to objective scrutiny, meaning, suffering, pain and so on. But the dependence view, as we saw, is explicitly non-reductionist and so need not embrace a view in which persons are regarded as objects.

So we can agree with Benner and Wrubel that it is mistaken to view persons as objects, and we can agree that a Cartesian line is one which should be rejected. But positions other than that put forward by Merleau-Ponty embrace the commitments Benner and Wrubel favour here. It is not only Merleau-Ponty's position which rejects the view of persons as objects. A non-reductionist 'dependence view' such as that described above offers support for such a line.

Second, with regard to the 'embodied intelligence' issue, it is clear how a reductionist view seems inadequate here. Intelligence seems a mental (or at least non-physical) property, yet reductionist positions must claim it is physical. Of course, so-called 'computer models of the mind' may be invoked to persuade us that this really is the case. But let us set this possibility aside. What does seem clear is that, once again, the 'dependence view' appears not to exclude the idea of embodied intelligence. The reason is, recall, within this view, mental properties such as intelligence can be conceived of as properties of physical things, for example human bodies. So if what is meant by 'embodied intelligence' is a property of a human body, then the dependence view is compatible with ideas of such intelligence – know-how. So acceptance of this idea need not lead us straight to Merleau-Ponty.

Third, a complex of related considerations were grouped under this discussion. But the two main elements focused on cognition and the nature of the person. The Cartesian picture of the person presented by Benner and Wrubel is of a detached reasoner, coolly evaluating her options. The information is provided to the mind by the senses. By contrast, the Merleau-Pontian view regards the person as a 'creature of significance' (1989, p. 52); immersed within a culture and inseparable from cultural elements such as language and other social practices.

Let us suppose the Cartesian picture of the detachable person is objectionable. The person, it may be said, is at least partly constituted by language and social phenomena. The Merleau-Pontian line certainly endorses a view such as this. But so too does the dependence view, especially since this is often linked with positions which are anti-Cartesian. (See the position known as externalism. In this, at least some mental phenomena are held to be dependent upon the existence of social and physical realms (McGinn, 1982; Macdonald, 1990; Edwards, 1994).)

With regard to the 'cognition' element of Cartesianism, again I can see no reason why this cannot be accommodated within a non-Cartesian, but also non-Merleau-Pontian position.

The upshot, then, is that Benner and Wrubel's championing of Merleau-Pontian line omits to consider a non-reductionist option which lies between, so to speak, those two positions. The position appears to have the benefits which Benner and Wrubel attribute to Merleau-Ponty's view, and also avoids the aspects of Cartesianism which they reject.

As seen, the dependence view is not without problems, for example concerning mind–body causation, but these may not be insuperable. The Merleau-Pontian line can sound attractive but it too has difficulties, such as those mentioned earlier in criticism of it. And, significantly, in that it requires a revision of the language within which we discuss what we currently term 'mental' and 'physical' phenomena. For on the Merleau-Pontian view, this is a mistake, it seems. So we seem to have a situation which is close to intractable. For what they are worth, here are some views of my own on this apparent stand-off.

One commentator on Merleau-Ponty's work, Dillon (1997, p. xviii), suggests that dualism is a phase within which western thought is currently locked. Our very language is replete with contrasts between the mental and the physical realms. These realms are interrelated, defined in terms of their contrast with one another. Dillon's suggestion is that this dualism is a hindrance to our ontological thinking, one which our philosophical thought will eventually break through and reformulate in other terms. According to Dillon the work of Merleau-Ponty will help to forge such a breakthrough.

One precondition to a development within ontology of such a kind would seem to be a breakdown in our existing ontology. Thus if it could be shown that the categories of the mental and the physical somehow do not do justice to the phenomena under study, then the need to develop and explore a radical new ontology is likely to become more pressing. I suspect that the philosophical examination of the phenomena of health care will prove important in such a development – that is, in a rejection of a dualism between the mental and physical realms. Phenomena such as pain, psychosomatic illness, mental illness, disability, and indeed embodied knowledge all seem to me to hold the key to breaking free of our current mode of conceptualising 'mental and physical' phenomena.

However, these are just thoughts on my part. The breakdown in our current mode of thinking has not yet been shown compelling. Thus at present, it seems to me that to favour the Merleau-Pontian line over the dependency view is the less satisfactory option: less satisfactory because it is the most radical. Quinean dictates relating to theory choice indicate preferences for current theory, as long as it is relatively successful. On the assumption that this can indeed still be said of our division between the mental and the physical it is proposed here that the dependence view is a more favourable basis within philosophy of mind than is the Merleau-Pontian rival. It is suitably anti-Cartesian and does not require the radical revision required by subscription to the Merleau-Pontian position. (Recall our virtues of conservatism and modesty in theory choice here.)

Evaluation

To try now to take stock of all four of the positions we have considered. Although all four positions have problems, it seems reasonable to suggest that two of them are so problematic that we can set them aside. The view which reduces the mental component of persons to the physical component – type identity theory – seems very problematic indeed. In fact brief consideration of its application to the health care sphere can bring out even further the serious limitations of this position. Since the position reduces persons to wholly physical things, the type identity thesis implies that all health problems are also physical. Similarly, all treatments will be physical treatments. All health care needs will derive from deviations from normal functioning of physiological systems. More problematically, in this position, the question of whether or not a person is ill, and the severity of the illness, will be determined exclusively from the third person perspective. 'Legitimate' illnesses will stand in need of objective confirmation, hence the person's own view of the matter can be wholly sidelined as irrelevant.

The position has no difficulty in explaining how physical treatments for psychological problems are effective, but can it explain the effectiveness of psychological treatments, so-called 'talking cures' and so on? Here the direction of causation seems to be mind-to-body rather than body-to-brain.

This position also implies that psychiatric medicine is, in fact, simply part of neurology, for, if all illnesses and diseases are physical, so too are 'mental' illnesses, since the mental simply is the physical. So psychiatric medicine is now simply subsumed under general medicine. Similarly, all disabilities will be physical disabilities; thus, intellectual and sensory disabilities will simply be physical disabilities on this account.

These implications of the adoption of this view of persons help to illustrate its crucial weakness. This lies in the attempt to make public that which is essentially private: the experience of illness, and other kinds of mental experience.

The second position which we can set aside as being excessively problematic is Cartesian dualism, the position, surprisingly, which is actually endorsed by two contemporary nurse theorists (Watson and Holden). The difficulty here is that although persons may have minds, these simply do not seem separable from bodies in the way in which dualism claims.

Applied to the health care domain, the view implies that health problems can presumably arise in either mind or body, as can health needs. But the real problem for this account lies in explaining the efficacy of physical treatments. If the mind is separate from the body how can the effects of, for example, tranquillisers be explained? Also, how can conditions such as dementia be explained? This seems close to an untenable position.

In the light of the weaknesses of these two accounts of the person we will henceforth set them aside. However, as seen, each of the two remaining accounts has its problems. Although these are not so serious as the problems which beset the two positions we have set aside, they are still significant.

Applied to the health care domain, acceptance of the Merleau-Pontian position entails that the mental/physical illness/disability distinction is a myth. Health care needs and treatments will similarly be conceptualised in such a way that they are neither purely physical nor purely mental. Thus, on this line, all illnesses have inextricable physical and mental components, and so too do all disabilities. Similarly, all treatments will focus on both dimensions, physical and mental. It is no surprise that those nurse theorists who favour 'holistic' approaches to nursing and to the person are sympathetic to this position. Moreover, adoption of the Merleau-Pontian line would seem to demand radical revision of our conception of health care and of facilities, education and training. The division of nurse training into general and mental health branches would, for example, require wholesale revision. It would be predicated upon a distinction which is rejected by the Merleau-Pontian position.

The 'dependence view' is plainly a much less radical option. On this, health problems and needs stem from physical or psychological domains. Treatment, would seem to be either physical or psychological also. Hence, on this view, psychiatric medicine could preserve some degree of autonomy since the mental, although dependent upon the physical, would not be considered reducible to it. And the same can be said of disabilities: that is, these can be physical, or intellectual (although where would sensory disabilities be categorised? as physical or mental?).

Similarly, needs would be physical or mental. And since the mental is not reducible to the physical, there would still be a place for subjective phenomena such as feelings of illness and so on.

The conclusion advanced earlier is that considerations of modesty and conservatism (recall Quine and Ullian: 'the lazy world is the likely world') militate in favour of the dependency view above the Merleau-Pontian line. Both anchor mental phenomena in the physical domain (though the Merleau-Pontian will resist this mode of expression), and they each respect the strong intuition that we have a distinctive kind of access to our own experiences. Hence both approaches meet these key conditions of satisfactory theory. And with reference to nursing, neither approach entails the kind of reductive view of patients fostered by type identity theory.

What I intend to do next is describe a narrative conception of the person. This will be seen to be compatible with either a slightly modified dependence view or indeed a Merleau-Pontian position. We will then see how a narrative conception of the person is of vital importance to the nursing context.

5 Nursing the person (ii): the individual person as a narrative

We noted in the last section that persons seem to have both mental and physical characteristics or properties. However, we saw further that providing a satisfactory account of the way these aspects of a person are related is extremely problematic. We saw, finally, that two views of their relations seem plausible, although neither is without difficulties; these are the 'dependence view', and the view espoused by Merleau-Ponty. For reasons given in the last chapter, the former is being accepted here. But it should be added that much of what is claimed in this chapter is perfectly compatible with the adoption of a Merleau-Pontian position.

A narrative conception of the person

So far, then, we have said a little concerning the question of what constitutes a person (that is, separable mind and body? mental and physical properties? body only? and so on). But we have neglected the question of what makes it the case that a person is the same person from one time to a later or from an earlier time. This problem, the problem of personal identity, is one which has generated a tremendous amount of literature (for example Shoemaker and Swinburne, 1984; Parfit, 1986; Dennett, 1981). It is not necessary for us to consider very carefully all the proposals which have been advanced. Two main approaches are typical. The first focuses on psychological continuity. In this, continuity in one's mental life (memories, experiences) is both a necessary and a sufficient condition for personal identity. The second approach focuses on physical continuity in which possession of the same body is a necessary and a sufficient condition for personal identity. It is fair to say that, generally, both approaches lapse into 'brain possession' theories in which continued possession of the same brain is a necessary and a sufficient condition for personal identity. Roughly speaking, this is for the reason that psychological continuity is thought to require possession of the same brain, and to proponents of physical continuity theory the brain has seemed the most important body part.

Hence in both approaches the body – apart from the brain – is not considered central to personal identity. It is fair to say that many philosophers have been unhappy with such a conclusion, and that the problem of personal identity is not widely considered to have been solved.

In recent years a so-called narrative view of the person has emerged which is not without difficulties, but which accords with many intuitions concerning personal identity. For example, intuitions that make one the person one is, are the life one actually leads, the values which one tries to aspire to and respect, and the goals one tries to achieve. It is also a view in which the body has a central role. It is a view which has particular relevance to nursing and to health care more generally. Further, it is a view of personal identity which can sit with both the Merleau-Pontian position described in the previous section; and with the (slightly modified) dependence view described earlier. The relevant modification for the latter simply involves extending the physical properties relevant to identity to include bodily and not merely neurophysiological properties; in other words, to include properties of the *person* as a whole.

The general claim that persons can be characterised in terms of a narrative is put forward as follows by MacIntyre. He writes of:

> [A] concept of a self whose unity resides in the unity of a narrative which links birth to life to death as narrative beginning to middle to end (1985, p. 205; also Schectman, 1996).

The proposal is, then, that just as a narrative has a beginning, a middle and an end, so too does a human life. Further, in a narrative the phases of it are linked: there is a relationship of intelligibility between the phases; present events are related to past events and a story can be told which unifies the past and the present. Again, these features of narratives seem applicable to human lives. Thus consider a person such as Margaret Thatcher. Her life began in Grantham, in modest economic circumstances. She went to university, married, became an MP, leader of the Conservative Party, and then Prime Minister. In relating these details of her life we are following a temporal order, from beginning to later phases. Since she is still alive, the narrative of her life is not yet complete. Yet, of course, we could relate mini-narratives within that overall narrative, for example the story of her becoming Prime Minister of the UK. In relating such a story we would be describing how one phase of her life led to a later phase, how some actions and events related to subsequent and prior actions and events. Thus, for example, had not Edward Heath been deposed as leader of the Conservatives, Thatcher might not have become leader, and then PM and so on.

The life of a human person standardly involves actions undertaken by the person. Each act itself has a beginning, middle and end. Thus making a cup of tea begins with the intention to do so, and ends with the tea. Such acts are undertaken in a context which provides a background against which actions performed are assessable as rational or otherwise. So, for example, making the tea can be explained by reference to one's feeling thirsty or wishing to relax, or both. Alternatively, a series of actions such as sitting exams can be explained and made intelligible by reference to the context of education. A person's decision to sit exams can be made sense of by reference to their intention to become a nurse. Their intention to become a nurse can be made sense of by reference to the person's broader aims, say to help others, or earn money for a more comfortable life.

Such goals are imbued with value in that they reflect what is valued by the person concerned, for example helping others, leading a comfortable, pleasant life, and so on. Mini-narratives describing the sitting of exams, say, are thus to be made sense of by reference to the person's broader goals. These stem from and expose just what the person values.

We might usefully describe the pursuance of these broader goals in terms of an attempt to pursue a 'self-project', for example, this may be to become a good nurse, or a good footballer, or a good father and so on (I borrow the term from van Hooft, 1995). The narrative which serves to identify one can then be understood to be a description of the pursuance of a self-project. This amounts, as we heard, to a description of a life story. It should be added that the taking of a particular self-project appears centrally related to a self-conception. This is a view of the kind of person one aspires to be. One's self-project can be understood as an attempt to realise one's self-conception. This will also be imbued with value since it presupposes a view on a 'kind of person' that one considers it 'good' to be.

So it can be seen that day-to-day acts are narratival in form in the sense that they have a beginning, middle and end. Such acts nest within a self-project, which in turn nests within a self-conception, for example according to which one sees oneself as a particular kind of person – a nurse or a good person. The description of all this, amounts to one's narrative.

The whole narrative can be said to exemplify a unity in that the actions which comprise it are undertaken by a person with a particular perspective upon the events which comprise the narrative. This is the case since the narrative is shaped by actions on the part of the person and these stem from the particular perspective of the person, and involve attempts on their part to bring about or respond to situations.

It should be stressed also that *interpretation* is evidently an important component of the narrative conception of the person. For the overall goals at which one aims presuppose an *interpretation* of the kind of person which one wants to be, or which one takes oneself to be. So one's 'self-conception' inevitably involves an interpretation of just what kind of person one wants to be. And in pursuing this in one's self-project, interpretation is inevitable in that actions are interpreted by the actor in relation to the self-conception of the person. For example, taking exams will presumably be explicable within a person's narrative, in that the person concerned takes it to be the case that passing the exams makes it more likely that they will become the kind of person they aspire to be. And also the day-to-day actions which comprise mini-narratives presuppose some interpretation of the relations between these acts and 'where one is aiming to get in life' so to speak.

In fact, the prevalence of interpretation is evident throughout our existence as a human person. Thus, for example, when entering a room full of people we interpret their responses to us as friendly, unfriendly, puzzled and so on. And mundane acts such as buying a newspaper from a shop presuppose interpretations such that the shop is the appropriate kind for the purchase of newspapers, and interpretations concerning the kinds of acts which are appropriate to effect such a purpose. One's day-to-day acts can be seen as constitutionally involving interpretations, and these in turn are bound to a view of the kind of person one is or is aiming to be. Each of these suppose interpretations on the part of the person since they presuppose interpretations of some ways of living as preferable to others, and some kinds of persons as preferable to others. Thus Benner and Wrubel (1989) (following Taylor (1985)), refer to persons as 'self-interpreters'. Their actions stem from interpretations of situations, and from conceptions of the kinds of persons they wish to be, the kinds of goals they wish to meet and aim for.

A note needs to be made here concerning the role of the third person perspective in the narrative account of the person. MacIntyre asserts 'I am what I may justifiably be taken by others to be' (1985, p. 217); and also 'we are never more than the co-authors of our own narratives' (ibid., p. 213). These brief remarks help to emphasise the weight accorded to the third person perspective in the narrative line. The concepts which shape or frame a narrative include those such as nationality, family membership, employment, and leisure interests. These are concepts applicable from the third person perspective and constrain one's own account of who one is.

Thus suppose I claim to be Brazilian yet there is no evidence of this, and there is plenty of evidence to the contrary – perhaps my family all point out that I was born in Salford, as they were. Further, there is no evidence that I or anyone else likely to have conceived me has any connection whatsoever with Brazil. Surely, as MacIntyre implies, I cannot plausibly claim to be Brazilian, while they can 'justifiably' deny that I am. Hence, there is a role for evidential considerations in the specification of narratives.

By the claim that 'we are never more than the co-authors of our own narratives' (ibid., p. 213) MacIntyre seems to mean, in effect, that the world resists and constrains our own self-projects and self-conceptions. Hence, I may wish at this moment that I am a millionaire and plan what I would do – say, become widely known as a rich benefactor of some worthy cause. However, of course I am not a millionaire, cannot enact my plans and so cannot acquire the reputation of a rich philanthropist. Thus I can never be the 'sole author', as MacIntyre puts it, of the narrative that describes me, my identity.

In fact, the third person perspective functions as a constraint upon narratives since many (perhaps all) of the concepts employed by subjects in their intentional states (beliefs, desires) will be derived from the social context they inhabit. For example the very idea of a person feeling embarrassed presupposes the presence of other people and of certain social norms of behaviour since the concept of embarrassment makes sense only given other people and relevant social conventions (Taylor, 1985).

It should be added that bodily appearance is also plausibly regarded as a key structuring component within the narratives of human persons. The way we appear affects the way in which others interact with us and also the way we interact with them – I mean to include our clothing, posture, facial expressions and so on as included within our bodily appearance. In wearing a uniform, in looking like a young child or an adult, or a very old frail person, the way we appear to others inevitably has an effect upon the way they interact with us. The pursuance of one's self-project inevitably involves the recognition of and response to this.

In summary then, according to a narrative conception of the identities of persons, a person's identity is constituted by a narrative. This is a description of a self-project. And a self-project is driven by a self-conception; the latter are inevitably imbued with value. The narratives which constitute identity respect intuitions regarding the centrality of the first-person perspective in accounts of the person in that a crucial role is accorded to persons' own interpretations of events. But narratives are also constrained from the third-person perspective, first by evidential considerations of the kind described above, and second by the linguistic and other social conventions which in part determine the interpretations of the person.

Two clarifications

Before moving on to show how this approach to personal identity applies in relation to nursing practice, I would like, first, to make two clarifications of it in order to avoid, as much as possible, any misunderstandings. Then I will say a little about the idea of *narrative understanding.*

First, it is being proposed here that the identities of persons can be conceived of in terms of a narrative. Each person will have a distinct narrative due to the fact that no two persons can lead identical lives. This is trivially true in that no two people occupy the same spatio-temporal locations throughout their lives, or even once in their lives. I can never experience the world from exactly the same position as another person.

Second, it is not being claimed here that persons *are* (literally are, are identical with) narratives. This is an implausible view in my opinion (but see Kerby (1991); Ricoeur (1992)). To see why, recall the logical rule which served as a constraint on identity relations in our discussion of the mind–body problem (Chapter 4). This held that if two things are identical, they must share all properties. Consider, then, persons and narratives.

Evidently, a narrative can commence even prior to conception. A childless couple may plan to have a child, discuss which university they will attend, which school and so on. This planning may continue after the child is conceived and beyond. But the point is that the narrative appears to precede the existence of the child. Thus, persons and narratives cannot be identical. Similarly, the narrative of a person seems not to end with their death. The narrative of Robert Maxwell, the media tycoon, continued well after his death, and was radically revised in the face of facts which came to light only after it. Again, this shows that persons cannot be identical to narratives. And of course, the idea of having a self-project emerges well after birth. It may even be the case that persons and narratives belong to differing ontological categories. But I will not pursue that here. The purpose of these last remarks has been to quash any suggestion that it is being claimed here that persons are narratives. What is being claimed is that the identities of persons can be understood as captured by a narrative, that which describes one's life story.

The final remarks to be made in this section concern the idea of *narrative understanding*. Given that we have a grasp of the idea that the identities of persons can be conceived of in narrative terms, it can be proposed further that understanding persons requires some conception of their narrative. This understanding we can term narrative understanding. Thus in trying to work out why a person acts in one way rather than in another we are engaged in the task of narrative understanding of the person. That is, we are trying to make sense of their actions in terms of their relations to the person's self-project.

To take a fairly straightforward example, in his recent autobiography *Managing My Life*, Alex Ferguson explained why he encouraged the sale of a player, Paul Ince, who seemed to outsiders to be a key element to the team's success. From Ferguson's perspective, Ince could no longer be relied upon to follow his tactical instructions, and in the light of this, was a liability rather than an asset to the team.

So here we are engaged in the process of understanding Ferguson's action, specifically, why he chose to sell Ince rather than keep him at the club. This mini-narrative (the circumstances surrounding the sale of Ince), is nested within Ferguson's larger narrative, a key structuring concept of which is the goal of success in football management at the highest level. Aspects of this larger narrative provide the context against which the decision to sell Ince is a rational one. Not selling him, as far as Ferguson is concerned, makes it less rather than more likely that he (Ferguson) will attain the goals which motivate him and that his self-project will be realised. Hence here we have an example in which understanding an action requires understanding of the narrative of the person.

We can contrast narrative understanding as just described with other kinds of understanding, for example biological understanding. If we take this to involve descriptions of humans in purely physical terms, it is unlikely that much understanding of human action will prove possible. For, given that actions are explained by mental phenomena, and that such phenomena are not reducible to physical phenomena, it follows that explanations of action in purely physical terms will not provide narrative understanding. And it is this which seems most central to understanding why persons act in the ways they do.

The significance of this will be evident in the next section when we look at the implications for practice of these claims. For ultimately the significance of the phenomena of health, disease and illness turns out to be inseparable from narrative-bound considerations. In short, the significance of these phenomena (health and so on) is inseparable from the significance attached to them by persons in terms of their self-projects.

Nursing and the narrative view of the person

It is time now to consider further how these claims relating to narrative identity bear upon nursing practice. The adoption of a narrative account of the individual person has a number of implications for nursing care. Specifically, it suggests that in order to understand a person, to understand what they say and do, it will be necessary to place what they say and do within the context of their narrative. The term 'narrative understanding' was invoked to characterise this mode of understanding.

We will also see in this section that narrative understanding has a place in the nursing care of patients even where there is no apparent first-person perspective present. For example, the view that narrative has an important place within nursing has implications for the way in which seriously cognitively impaired humans and human foetuses are viewed. In addition, as we will see in this section, it has implications for the idea of health promotion, and the understanding of mental health problems.

As noted in the previous section, narratives are by definition continuous. This continuity is temporal, but is not just that. Relations of intelligibility hold between earlier and later stages of a narrative. We noted further that typically there are first- and third-person perspectives on narratives, and that in most cases a narrative is a combination of what is told from each of these perspectives.

With reference to the relevance of narrative understanding in the health care context, this helps to account for the *significance* of illness. Persons are engaged in a series of actions which are the mini-narratives the description of which constitute their larger narrative. Illness poses a threat to the pursuance of a narrative. Illness may prevent one from engaging in acts which one views as central to one's self-project. It might prevent one from competing in or training for a sporting event, or attending a family celebration, or parenting in the way in which one wishes to, or even working. So the significance of illness can be seen to be tied to a person's self-project. Narrative understanding in nursing involves the attempt to see the significance of patients' descriptions of symptoms in terms of their self-projects.

To take another example, recall the case of the professional dancer referred to at the beginning of Chapter 4, Introduction. Dancing is a key concept, what we may term a structuring concept, within her narrative; that is to say, dancing is a central activity for that person, an activity in which much time is engaged, and in relation to which other activities are organised and prioritised.

This person's narrative centrally involves the activity of dancing. Given this, and given the person's strong desire to dance it is plain that any illness, believed by that person to impede her dancing career, will be a cause of great concern to her. The dancer interprets her symptoms in terms of her self-project. The suggestion is that it is important for the nurse to do so also.

Once the dancer experiences some symptoms which she takes to pose a threat to her dancing, then the level of concern this generates will be present regardless of whether *in fact* the symptoms do point to a health problem which will adversely affect her ability to dance. So it appears crucial to take into account a person's own interpretation of their symptoms and their likely effects upon their life. In caring for a person such as the dancer in a nursing context it seems extremely important and helpful to gather some sense of the patient's own view of their symptoms. For it is this interpretation which will affect their mood and behaviour during their time in the clinical setting (and of course before and after this). Awareness of such interpretations by the nurse seems, plausibly, to be useful in helping the patient to cope with their predicament. This is the case since, at least, the nurse can then become aware of the source of the patient's anxiety and be better equipped to deal with this appropriately.

The example suggests again that evaluating people's health problems solely in biological terms is inadequate. For it is the significance of the biological data for a particular patient which is crucial to the proper care of that person. Hence understanding of the person in biological terms needs to be supplemented with narratival understanding. As we have seen this involves trying to grasp the patient's conception of her symptoms. This conception will be in terms of the narrative of the patient, her values, goals and self-project.

These last paragraphs have been an attempt to show how appreciation of the narrative of a person is relevant to their nursing care.

Narratival understanding may also elucidate at least some of the causes of illness. This is due to the point that some narratives are associated with unhealthy lifestyle choices. Thus a lifestyle which involves heavy smoking, drinking and poor diet may be part of the narrative of certain groups of people. Just as for the dancer, dancing played a structuring role in her narrative, it may be that for a person, socialising in contexts inseparable from drinking and smoking is crucial for them. Thus, as with the dancer, it is socialising in relation to which all other activities are evaluated and prioritised.

So it seems easy to point to a close relationship between certain lifestyles and illness, and to conceptualise this relation in narrative terms. And, as with the dancer example, it seems important to try to obtain a view of a patient's narrative in order to try to understand the nature of their illness. Thus, for example, as will be discussed later, it is likely to be more difficult to change a pattern of behaviour which is associated with an important feature of a person's narrative, than one which is peripheral to a narrative.

Narratival understanding can be shown to be crucial to concepts such as suffering. A definition of it offered by Cassell runs thus: 'Suffering can be defined as the state of severe distress associated with events that threaten the intactness of the person' (1991, p. 33). His proposal here is that suffering involves not simply the experience of distress, but that a threat to the very intactness of the person is required. By 'intactness' Cassell means the capacity of a person to pursue their self-projects. Put another way, suffering is a direct consequence of a perceived threat to one's capacity to pursue a self-project.

Thus if a person experiences symptoms of ill-health, this is not yet sufficient for them to be suffering. Suffering only ensues if the person interprets these symptoms as posing a threat to their capacity to pursue what they most value. Thus if the most important thing in a person's life is dancing – if this is a structuring concept in their narrative – any symptoms which are thought by them to pose a threat to this may cause the person to suffer. The reason is that dancing is so central to that person's identity – to their self-project – that if they cannot dance, their very identity is under threat. Hence Cassell's use of the expression 'intactness'. In health, one is 'intact', one can pursue one's goals. The experience of certain kinds of symptoms of ill health causes suffering due to their placing in jeopardy values and goals which the person cherishes, which partly define who that person is.

Again it follows that mere biological understanding of a person will not reveal whether or not they are suffering. If Cassell is right, narratival engagement with the person is necessary to discern this.

Closely related points can be made in regard to equally central notions such as quality of life and health. A life of good quality can be assimilated to a life in which one can pursue what is important to one. This need not be thought synonymous with a happy life; it is plausible to suppose there to be more to leading a life of good quality than the mere experience of happiness. The pursuance of goals is rarely, if ever, accompanied by complete happiness. Rather it involves effort, some hardship and so on. These experiences contribute to make the achievement of goals satisfying. So the idea of narrative again can be seen to help explicate the idea of quality of life (see Benner, 1985).

With regard to health, as may be anticipated, on a narrative-oriented understanding of this, a person is healthy when they are not impeded (by factors internal to their bodies) from pursing that which is important to them, when they are able to pursue what Nordenfelt terms their vital goals (1995). Having made these general points concerning the place of narrative in nursing care, a further illustration of them will be made with reference to the mental health context.

Narrative and mental health problems

As with physical illness, mental illness can be seen in terms of a disruption in a person's narrative. Due to the illness the person becomes unable to pursue the goals which figure within their narrative. The impact of severe mental illness may be such that a person's life seems to have no discernible goals or plans. Or to lead to narratives which are bizarre or apparently incoherent. Of course these judgements concerning the intelligibility of a narrative are made from the third-person perspective. But this is legitimate within the narrative position. For, to recall MacIntyre, one cannot be the sole author of one's narrative. And relatedly, judgements concerning intelligibility and rationality are all bound to the social context within which the person is situated. So given the link between the concepts of mental illness and rationality, it is inevitable that a social aspect to such illnesses will be present.

This suggests mental illness cannot be understood without reference to the cultural context of a person. It is in relation to this that a person's narrative will be constructed, and constrained. This implies that great care is needed in diagnosing mental illness in people from cultures other than ones with which one is very familiar. For the idea of narrative understanding requires such familiarity. Otherwise, there is a great risk of misunderstanding (see, for example, Kleinman, 1986).

Consider also a case not involving cultural differences but in which a person's narrative takes a very significant change. For example, a person is a grandmother who takes a lively interest in her grandchildren, babysitting, taking them on outings and so on. In addition, although not in paid employment, the person has a lively social life and sees the maintenance of the home as a key part of her role, her self-project. Thus the house is regularly cleaned and kept tidy. Gradually, the grandmother appears to lose interest in her grandchildren, even refusing to allow them in her house, without any apparent reason. The house itself becomes shabby; she no longer cleans it. And the socialising also stops; the grandmother rarely leaves the house. The family notice these dramatic changes. They do not seem to be the kinds of changes which make sense; in other words, narrative understanding of them is problematic given the values evident in the person's previous actions (for example of commitment to grandchildren, a clean house and so on). The family, concerned, alert the person's GP. She arranges for a CPN to visit the grandmother. The CPN detects no discernible mental health problems. Upon speaking to the grandmother, she answers the CPN's questions satisfactorily ('how are you?' 'Do you know your family are concerned about your health? and so on). The CPN leaves and assumes the woman's family are unnecessarily alarmed. The family, however, remain convinced the woman is unwell.

One reason for giving great weight to the views of close relatives in a situation of this kind can be explained by reference to the idea of narratival understanding. The family have a greater appreciation of the gap between the person's previous acts and her current patterns of acting. The former patterns of action clearly fit within an intelligible narrative. But, at least for them, the recent actions fit into no coherent narrative. There seems no explanation for the change in actions, and no intelligible direction or coherence to the pattern of acts currently undertaken by the grandmother.

What seems to be the case here, is that the close family have a more adequate narrative understanding of the plight of the grandmother than the CPN. For, it seems reasonable to claim, the question of whether or not the person has a mental health problem cannot be answered without reference to that person's overall narrative. A sense of the nature of this cannot be obtained within the scope of a brief interview of the kind conducted (hypothetically) in the meeting between the CPN and the grandmother. And the general claim can be made to the effect that diagnosing mental illness requires narrative understanding of the person whose illness is in question. (Needless to add, this may not be possible to obtain, for example if the person refuses to speak to the relevant health care professional.)

Once again, these points bring out the poverty of an understanding of mental illness in purely physical terms. For it is only when acts are described at the intentional level that such illness becomes apparent. (For further references regarding narrative-based medicine, see for example Kleinman, 1988; Greenhalgh and Hurwitz, 1998.) Consider now the idea of narrative understanding in relation to health promotion.

Health promotion

Benner and Wrubel draw attention to the illusory nature of the idea of total or 'radical' freedom (1989, p. 23; also Parse, 1998). On the narrative view of the person, since persons are always enmeshed within a narrative, they are 'free' in a qualified sense only. The kinds of options which seem attractive or even possible for a person will be determined in part by their past. Thus for example in the earlier part of the 20th century in the UK entry to university was common for (male) 18-year-olds within some socio-economic groups, and very uncommon for 18-year-olds from lower socio-economic groups. It is reasonable to suppose that 'going to university' would figure routinely in the planned self-projects of the former group but not for the latter.

And of course the freedom persons have is constrained by several factors. These include the person's values, and the obligations the person has, for example to relatives, friends, and employers. Also included are the sedimented habits which contribute to the distinctive identity of the person – for example being a 'nervous' edgy person, being a chain smoker, being a serious person, or being lighthearted, being adapted to having a chronic illness, and so on.

As Benner and Wrubel state:

> [Persons] enter into situations with their own sets of meanings, habits and perspectives. And the particular ways of being in the situation set up particular lines of action and possibilities. New possibilities can be learned, but they are encountered or introduced only in the context of the old habits, skills, practices and expectations (1989, p. 23).

Much of this is in accord with a narrative conception of the identities of persons. Consider the implications of this account for the giving of health advice. Suppose a life-long smoker and heavy drinker complains of symptoms of heart disease. The nurse advises the person to stop smoking and drinking. It is not likely that the person will simply be able to change his unhealthy lifestyle immediately; that would involve a radical disjunction in the person's narrative. The scale of the change in behaviour that is being prescribed by the nurse is close to a change in identity for that person, assuming that the person is a chain smoker, say. The habits sedimented over a lifetime cannot simply be changed overnight.

It is tempting to observe that these are truisms: of course people cannot change overnight. But what is being suggested here is that these truths are grounded in a particular view of what it is to be the person one is. The view provides a philosophical foundation, and an explanation for the truism just identified, and the truism can be invoked in support of the philosophical account. Further, the truism can help to show the inadequacy of biological accounts of the person. Descriptions of persons in such terms omit the intentional level. Yet clearly it is in such intentional terms that the acts of persons are conceived of and described.

So applied to the health promotion context, the narrative account appears to imply that the kinds of health changes which it is possible for people to undergo need to be viewed within the context of their narrative. This narrative will expose the values and commitments held dear by the patient. Health advice must take this into account in order to have any chance of being acted upon by the patient.

Two further specific points. First, it seems to me to be a merit of the narrative account that it explains how people can come to view their disability or chronic illness as part of what it is to be them. Such conditions can come to dominate the person's life and so become a major structuring aspect of their narrative (see, for example Morris, 1991; Toombs, 1993; 1995).

Second, obtaining a patient's history is obtaining their narrative. Hence Benner and Wrubel (1989, p. 16) suggest that this is the first stage in nursing the person. Obtaining such a story will be crucial because the significance of the illness depends centrally upon the significance accorded to it by the patient – that is, depending upon the patient's interpretation of his symptoms. So proper nursing care depends upon appreciation of the patient's interpretation of his situation, and important clues to the nature of that interpretation are to be found in the illness-narrative told by the patient.

However, in some cases, the first-person perspective is either not yet developed (as in the foetus or neonate), is inchoate (for example as in dementia) or is absent altogether (for example in persistent vegetative state (PVS)). What can be said of such cases from the perspectives of narrative identity and understanding?

Dementia

Consider the care of people with dementia. Prior to the onset of the condition the person's identity is constituted in the usual way by their narrative. During the initial stages of the illness the character of the narrative changes due to the effects of the illness on the first-person perspective of the narrative; that is, due to the adverse effects of the dementia on the cognitive capacities of the person. Gradually, the integrity of the first-person perspective erodes.

The appeals to narrative as comprising identity, and to narrative understanding appear to motivate specific ways of dealing with such people. For example, a focus on the narrative of the dementing person's life ensures that the person's condition is not viewed exhaustively in neurophysiological terms. Viewing persons with dementia in such terms has come under increasing criticism in recent years (especially. Kitwood, 1997). It is suggested that a focus on the neurological dimension of the condition generates a neglect of other strategies for caring for sufferers. A focus on the person's narrative, and on significant elements within it, can apparently help to redress the previous over-emphasis on neurological data, and to delay the progression of the condition (Kitwood, 1997). And of course such an emphasis helps to remind carers of the individuality of such patients, that they have led full lives, have families, occupations and hobbies and so on. This can serve an important role in protecting such individuals from being regarded as having a low moral standing by their carers, and arguably, can help to stave off the risk of neglect. If patients are 'anonymised' by a regime of care, it is plausible to suppose the level of care to be inferior to regimes in which care is focused on the individual as a person. Attention to the narrative of the patient can help to preserve such a focus. In other words, strategies of care designed to prolong rather than erode narrative identity, prolong the scope for narrative understanding of the person.

It should be said again that a focus on the intentional level of human life as opposed to a focus on the physical level is supported by our rejection of the reductionist ('type identity') theory. This suggests there are good philosophical grounds to suppose that persons are essentially such that they are describable in intentional terms (for example in the terms of narratives) as opposed to being essentially describable in purely biological terms. For what is most important about persons is that which is described at the intentional level. It is at this level of discourse that the things which matter to personal identity are couched (that is, one's name, values, relationships and so on).

Moreover, recall the requirement that narratives be continuous and intelligible. These relations of intelligibility indicate that narratives cannot standardly be 'fractured' or exhibit radical contingency. To give an extreme example of such a limit, the narrative of a person cannot transform into that of a frog. Consider the person whose mental condition has deteriorated to such an extent that he requires institutional care. The person's own grasp on their narrative is highly tenuous. Presumably, in the person's own home environment that grasp will be continually prompted by significant clues, for example a picture of a spouse, a treasured ornament, perhaps a pet. In this context, the narrative is still continuous in a sense which is more than simply temporal.

Removing the person from this home environment seems, plausibly, to pose a threat to the person's narrative. One way to ease the transition, and to ensure that the transition is not disjointed or 'fractured' would seem to be to surround the person with as many familiar things as possible, and to reduce, as much as possible, the strangeness of the new environment. Of course, this is hardly a new innovation in care practice. But it shows how the narrative view of the identity of persons applies in practice.

PVS patients

The first-person perspective in cases of persistent vegetative state (PVS) is reportedly absent. We are told that such people have irreversibly lost the very capacity for conscious thought and even sensation. Thus in such cases there is no question of the pursuance by the patient of a self-project. Although this may previously have been true of the person in PVS, it is not now.

Yet it is reported that nurses caring for such people 'construct' narratives for them: speaking to them about things that were of interest to them prior to their developing PVS, for example football, music, friends and so on (de Raeve, 1996).

Hence, as with the person with dementia, the person in PVS remains embedded in a network of relations, and within a network of narratives. (The patient is a subject of a narrative, but not of experience.) However, given the ontology of persons described above (Chapter 4) in which persons are beings with both mental and physical properties, it seems to follow that the status of humans in PVS as persons is called into question. I suspect there is no option other than to accept this. However certain important qualifications need to be made concerning precisely what such a view entails.

It is worth making explicit that the claim that humans in PVS are no longer persons is an ontological claim. No claims regarding the moral standing of such patients are entailed by this. The further question of whether such patients should be thought to have the same moral standing as persons is not one we need to take on. But it is important to stress that the ontological claim concerning the lack of personhood of humans in PVS, by itself, does not generate any particular normative conclusions regarding the moral standing of such patients.

Indeed, as we have seen, what seems to happen in such cases is that carers and relatives construct narratives for such patients, and these are related to the earlier narrative of the patients. Also, given that the patient in PVS typically did once have a self-project, one wonders what the ontological force of this might be, that is, could it count in favour of including humans in PVS within the category of persons? (A remark of Kerby's is striking here. He suggests that the human body is a 'site of narration' (1991, p. 4)).

It is well known that the moral standing of patients in PVS has been contested. For the properties necessary for personhood, according to many influential views (for example Harris, 1985), are lost irrevocably in this condition. In terms of narrative identity it is claimed that since the first-person perspective is irreversibly absent, the moral standing of the individual is thereby reduced. Yet, as we have seen, this normative claim is certainly not entailed by the ontological claim.

Before moving on to say something about the human foetus, it is worth signalling a difference between foetuses on the one hand, and the patient with dementia or PVS on the other. It seems clear that in the latter two cases their narratives are well-established – sedimented, as it may be put. The narratives of such people acquire a constancy and a character over time; their characteristics accrete to form a kind of unity. As noted, this will be a unity of intelligibility which stretches back in time from the origin of the person concerned. This temporal element of narrative, this sedimentation, is absent in the case of the foetus.

The human foetus

It can seem plausible to claim that foetuses have a narrative. Given the lack of clarity over the cognitive function of foetuses it is not clear that there is much of a first-person perspective to the narrative of the foetus. Yet it is clear that third-person considerations are present in the construction of the narrative of the person. The narrative of the foetus may even have begun prior to conception. Perhaps the parents are desperate for a child and imagine what he or she would be like. Or, they may be undergoing a process of assisted conception. It is reasonable to suppose that the narrative of the foetus thus begins prior to birth and possibly also even prior to conception.

With reference to nursing care, it seems that viewing the foetus in narrative terms renders it more likely that the nurse or midwife will view the foetus with a significance which is bound to and derives from its relationship to its parent(s). Again, this militates against a view of the foetus in purely biological terms.

Finally, with reference to the nursing care of humans in which a first-person perspective is absent, it should be said that it remains true of such patients that they have what we can term a 'plight'. By this I mean to refer to the morally salient features of their predicament. Such salient features may relate to prolonged experience of pain, or discomfort, or in the case of PVS patients, to the sense of a tragedy which has befallen them. The idea of a plight, thus signals the fact that persons are the kinds of things which can suffer, and which have a past, and a present which is oriented to the future (recall our remarks concerning the idea of a self-project). So the idea of an individual's having a plight draws attention to the fact that human lives are not to be conceived of as a 'snapshot'. As such it is an idea parasitic upon the notion of narrative understanding.

The idea of a plight is a broad notion which can apply to all humans. It signals the idea that there are likely to be morally salient features of the situation in which a human finds themselves which strike those caring for them. It has been said here that such a notion applies to the care of PVS patients, but it plainly applies across to other patients too, and this is an idea we return to in our discussion of care below (Chapter 6).

In the present section we have attempted to articulate the relevance of a narrative conception of the person to nursing. In this, recall, a narrative is a description of the pursuance of a self-project. Given that the idea of pursuance of a self-project is applicable only after infancy, it is clear that narratives can commence prior to the emergence of a self-project. It is when such a project develops that the idea of a distinctive identity takes hold.

At the other end of life, a narrative may continue when the capacity to pursue a self-project is lost, notably in PVS and even in death. So plainly narrative can continue beyond the loss of pursuance of a self-project.

The narrative conception of the person applies least problematically to the care of those with a self-project. But note that adoption of this idea does not entail that the nursing care of those patients without a self-project cannot be made sense of. Clearly, such patients have a plight. And nursing care represents a proper response to this.

We now turn to discuss a problem with the narrative conception of the person even as it applies in the least problematic cases (that is, those able to pursue a self-project).

Criticism of the narrative conception of the person: the contingency of narratives

As seen in Chapter 1 above a distinction can be drawn between contingent and necessary features of things. In our discussion of the relations between mental and neurological states it was argued that there is only a contingent relationship between any particular mental event M, and any particular neurological event N. If the relationship between N and M is indeed contingent, it follows that N could have occurred without M occurring, and M could have occurred without the occurrence of N – that is, since N is no part of the nature of M, is not reducible to M.

With reference to persons it is common, again, to distinguish contingent and necessary features of them. So, suppose one wants to describe those features, *those properties*, of a person which uniquely distinguish *that* person from others. Suppose in doing so one observes that a person has just lost a single hair. This is not likely to lead us to the belief that the person is literally a different person. Some properties of persons seem not to be relevant to their identities – to be contingent to their identity – and others seem to be necessary. Thus in attempting to identify the features which uniquely identified Florence Nightingale, one is more likely to point to her being female than to her being (say) 5'10" rather than 5'9". Of course, in order to get at those properties of Florence Nightingale which distinguished her from other females one would need to add considerably more details.

The attempt to point to those properties of persons which uniquely identify them thus exploits a distinction between contingent properties – roughly those which *are not* essential to the identity of the person in question; and necessary ones – roughly those which *are* essential to the identity of the person in question.

A criticism of the narrative conception of persons is that all properties of persons turn out to be contingent ones. In other words, any life a person actually leads could have been otherwise. Thus we mentioned Margaret Thatcher earlier. Any plausible narrative of her life must make reference to her being Prime Minister of the UK. Yet, had her early life been different, or had political circumstances been difficult she might not have become Prime Minister. It seems, thus, we can make sense of the idea of Margaret Thatcher not having become Prime Minister, of her life taking a different path, perhaps one consigned to the back benches, or even one outside politics altogether.

The criticism of the narrative conception is, then, that accounts of personal identity are required to identify those properties of a person which are necessarily true of them, those without which they would not be the person they are. Yet, the kinds of properties which figure in narratives, for example being Prime Minister, or being a nurse, or a teacher, or having a disability, or being tall and so on, all seem not to have this essential character. As the discussion of Mrs Thatcher's life shows, they all seem to be properties which are contingent, which a person might not have acquired had their life turned out differently.

Response

The criticism we identified concerned the contingency of the properties invoked in narrative accounts of the person. As outlined in Chapter 1 (in our discussion of two philosophical tools), there seems no option other than to accept this observation. In defence it may be claimed that the quest for essential properties of persons is in fact illusory. For all properties of persons are, in fact, contingent (see Rorty, 1989).

Having conceded this, two partial responses need to be made. First, although all characteristics are contingent some seem more central to a person's identity than others. For example a change in a person's gender seems a more radical change than losing a single hair or a tooth. Thus, borrowing the metaphor of a web from Quine once more, we might claim that characteristics at the 'centre' of the web are more crucial to personal identity than those at the periphery of the web. It is reasonable to suppose that gender would be one of those characteristics of a person which figures centrally, and not merely peripherally. For gender is likely to be crucial to a person's self-conception, and thus to the way they act, and also to the ways in which others respond to them.

(Recall the examples given earlier in this chapter of the dancer and the heavy smoker. These characteristics of these people are closer to the centre of their respective 'webs' than to the periphery.)

The second response seeks to identify some limits, of a formal nature, to this contingency. Thus for example, accounts of identity will be narratival in form, as will accounts of actions. Moreover, all narratives will be those of embodied individuals. All narratives will involve social elements, language, culture and so on. All narratives, by definition, involve appeal to spatio-temporal properties. These seem inescapable features of human narratives, and thus to present limits to the contingency mentioned in the criticism to which this is a partial response (see Smith, 1997).

In short, then, some formal features of narratives will be inevitable, for example relating to embodiment, to spatio-temporal categories and the narratival form itself. But how these are completed, so to speak, will be a contingent matter. For each individual narrative could have turned out otherwise. There seem reasonable grounds to grin and bear this philosophically: no successful theory of personal identity seems able to cope with the kinds of intuitions which point up contingency in narratives, and it does seem possible to posit some formal features of narratives. But further, and more important for present purposes, in dealing with people in the nursing context it is the details of a person's actual narrative which seem most pressing. It seems crucial to focus on the life the person is currently leading, as opposed to the life they might have lived. The example of the dancer discussed earlier clearly shows this. What is significant in nursing this person is the importance she attaches to being a dancer; this is in spite of the possibility that, had her life taken another course, she may not be so taken up with this activity.

Conclusions

We will now recap some of the points made in this chapter and the previous one and try to draw some general conclusions.

We began with Benner and Wrubel's observation that all theories of nursing presuppose some conception of the person. We then considered four main options in relation to this issue. We concluded that two of the four main theories could be rejected, and two others seemed plausible to varying degrees. After some consideration a 'dependency view' of the relations between mental and physical properties was put forward as the most favourable position within the theory of mind. Adoption of this entails a view of persons such that they have both mental and physical properties. And crucially, that the mental properties of thought, sensation and so on cannot be reduced to merely physical properties.

It is worth stressing that this seems a solid ontological foundation for the subsequent work on identity and narrative. It is also worth stressing that the dependency/token identity option appears not to be widely appreciated within nursing literature. Typically, once Cartesian dualism and a reductive type identity theory are dispensed with, the Merleau-Pontian position is presented as the sole option. As we have seen, this need not be the case.

With this 'dependency' position informing our understanding of persons we then considered the idea of the identities of persons as being constituted by a narrative. This seemed an especially important consideration in the nursing context. For in order to nurse a person it seems important to have some understanding of the significance which they attach to their own symptoms, and to their predicament generally; we characterised this as narrative understanding.

In the view of persons championed here, combined with a dependency view of relations between mental and physical states, persons are not identical to narratives, but their identities are constituted by their narratives: persons have narratives. This sits well with our adoption of the dependency view. For, as noted, in this we can conceive of persons as beings which have mental and physical properties, which have thoughts and feelings, and which have height, weight, and physical appearance. The narrative of a person serves to identify that person within the class of persons, and the properties employed to do this will be both mental and physical, for example comprising the person's aims, values, and other social phenomena, but not independent of their physical appearance. (Thus for example the narrative of a person with Down's syndrome is likely to include reference to the characteristic appearance of persons with that condition.)

All this is currently a summary of what has been claimed in this chapter. I would like now to spell out further some implications of this view of persons.

The account favoured here is a non-reductionist one, and one which thus holds that mental phenomena have aspects which cannot be captured in physical terms. Pain cannot be captured by (adequately described by) descriptions of any neurological phenomena thought to underlie it. It is defined, at least partially, by the way it feels. Pain has a crucial subjective element to it. The subjective element is crucial because it can be experienced only by the person undergoing it. Or, more strictly, pain cannot be experienced by any *other* person in the same way in which the person undergoing the experience of pain experiences it.

It follows that pain is, significantly, beyond the scope of medical science. By this it is meant that insofar as science requires that its data be open to public scrutiny, to be essentially publicly accessible, pain lies beyond it since it cannot, in principle, satisfy this requirement. Similar claims can be advanced with reference to any mental state the nature of which has a similarly crucial subjective element. Thus, suffering, well-being, quality of life, and perhaps health all have subjective aspects to them which are crucial to their natures.

Our brief discussion of mental health problems earlier also casts serious doubt on the prospect of understanding such problems solely in biological terms. For mental health problems themselves can only be understood and articulated in intentional terms. No purely biological description of a person (that is, in purely physical terms) will show that a person is mentally ill.

The discussion of narrative strongly suggests the centrality of this to an understanding of the person. And as noted the significance attributed to symptoms by patients depends in large measure on their perception of the impact of them upon their narrative. Since they seem best placed to judge this, or at least to be in a position of particular authority when it comes to making such a judgement, this again appears to generate serious problems for the project of medical science. For the significance attributed to symptoms by patients is not necessarily open to view. Again this has ramifications for the very possibility of scientific scrutiny of such data.

Moreover, consider that the very goals of health care will include reference to health, quality of life, best interests, and so on. Consider also that these appear best understood within the context of a person's narrative. Thus the question of what is in a person's best interests appears inseparable from that person's narrative. The dancer example given earlier suggests this. From the perspective of health care professionals it may be in the best interests of a person to refrain from dancing, for example due to the stress this exerts on the person (say, their heart, or joints, or both). But dancing may mean so much to the person, to have such a crucial place within their narrative, that they may judge continuing to dance to be in their best interests – even in spite of the warning from health care professionals that such a decision would not be in their best interests. I take it to be clear that exactly parallel considerations apply in relation to judgements regarding a person's quality of life. Their perspective on such questions seems a necessary one in such judgements, and seems especially authoritative (if not, perhaps, decisive).

This issue is illustrated well by consideration of the lives of people with disabilities. It is frequently judged that the quality of a life with disability is necessarily poor. Yet in many cases this conflicts with the view of the disabled person themselves. Surely the person's own judgement carries a particular authority. Within that person's own narrative they may be capable of doing all the activities they wish to.

These are issues to which we shall return in our discussion of the nature of nursing. For they seem to militate against the view of nursing as a science, that is, given that the data with which it is most centrally concerned appear to have this essentially personal aspect to them, to what extent are appeals to evidence-based practice and so on legitimate? One view is that they involve attempts to objectivise that which is essentially personal. Therefore, they are flawed in principle.

So far then, our epistemological enquiry in Chapters 2 and 3 led us to conclusions regarding the revisable nature of knowledge. Our ontological enquiry in Chapters 4 and 5 has led us to a specific conception of the person. It is one in which persons have both mental and physical properties, and in which their identities are described by a narrative. Given these claims within epistemology and ontology we move on to consider the topic of care. This will shed some light on the *moral* nature of nursing. As we will see, this moral nature of nursing can be shown to derive from two ontological features of humans: their vulnerability in the form of their capacity to experience pain and suffering, and second, their pursuance of a self-project. We will have cause to reconsider the idea of a 'plight' introduced in this chapter. As suggested above, it is a broad enough notion to be able to make sense of the idea of caring for others, even those without a self-project.

SUGGESTIONS FOR FURTHER READING

Texts on mind–body relations

As with knowledge, useful discussions on the relations between mind and body can be found in Nagel, Popkin and Stroll, and Grayling (with the reservation concerning difficulty noted above). Useful general introductions to this area include K. Campbell (1984) (2nd edn) *Body and Mind*, Notre Dame, Indiana: University of Notre Dame Press (this is brief and extremely clear); C. McGinn (1998) (2nd edn) *The Character of Mind*, Oxford: Oxford University Press (more difficult and perhaps 'deeper' than Campbell); and lastly R. Warner and T. Szubka (eds) *The Mind–Body Problem: A Guide to the Current Debate*, Oxford: Blackwell.

Persons

With regard to the topic of persons, a very useful text is P. Carruthers' (1989) book, *Introducing Persons*, London: Routledge.

Merleau-Ponty's work

Merleau-Ponty (1962) expresses his views but it should be said this is difficult reading. Helpful secondary literature includes M. Hammond, J. Howarth, and R. Keat (1991) *Understanding Phenomenology*, Oxford: Blackwell (Chapters 5, 6 and 7 provide a clear and accessible introduction to the work of Merleau-Ponty). A more difficult text is Stephen Priest (1998). See also Dillon (1997), and M.M. Langer (1989) *Merleau-Ponty's* Phenomenology of Perception, *A Guide and Commentary*, London: Macmillan – now Palgrave.

Narrative

On the idea of narrative applied to persons, Chapter 9 of B. Fay (1996) *Contemporary Philosophy of Social Science*, Oxford: Blackwell, is clear and useful. For lengthier discussions see Kerby (1991), Schectman (1996) and Ricoeur (1992), although each of these is hard going – the last mentioned especially.

6 Care in nursing (i): intentional care

This chapter and the next focus on the topic of care in nursing. The present chapter discusses the idea of intentional care; that is, care as involving a particular kind of mental attitude. Explication of this helps to bring out the moral nature of nursing. For nursing is best conceived of as a response to human vulnerability and suffering. Acts of intentional caring are inescapably involved in the nature of that response.

Our discussion commences with an examination of the idea of intentional care, and then moves on to consider the influential work on this topic undertaken by Noddings (1984). Following consideration of the relationship between emotion and care, we identify problems arising from the application of the idea of intentional caring to humans in persistent vegetative states, and to non-human animals. It is concluded, finally, that acts of intentional care within nursing require on the part of the nurse: a conception of the plight of the patient, a response to the patient's needs, and an 'emotional' component.

Intentional care[1]

The view that caring is central to or is the 'essence' of nursing is one which has received widespread attention and sympathy within nursing literature (for example Leininger, 1984; Watson, 1988). But it is often unclear just what is being claimed in such views. In extreme forms, it is claimed that caring is unique to nursing. For this strong view to be made out it would have to be shown that a form of caring existed which was undertaken solely by nurses. The focus of attempts to shore up such a 'uniqueness claim' is often the mental attitude of nurses performing such caring acts (for example Watson, 1988; Nortvedt, 1996). So articulation of such a version of the uniqueness claim would require the description of a kind of mental state which only nurses could adopt. This seems wildly implausible. Surely, doctors may care for their patients, parents for their children, social workers for their clients, and so on. Nonetheless, the view that caring is a concept related centrally to nursing does seem plausible. But even this more modest view is beset with problems: Do caring acts require a specific kind of 'mental attitude', perhaps including a specific kind of emotional 'involvement' with patients? If so, what would be the nature of this 'attitude'?

Matters have become still more complex by appeals to care in a new sense (new, at least, as far as nursing scholarship is concerned). This new sense appeals to an *ontological* sense of care, care as a way of 'being in the world' as it is said (Benner and Wrubel, 1989). This new sense is equally problematic and difficult to gain a clear understanding of.

The term 'caring' can be said of particular actions, persons and also professions. Hence the gentle reassurance of an anxious person, the person who undertakes that act, and her profession, can all be described as caring.

With reference to actions, it is common to claim that these stem from intentions to act on the part of the actor where intentions are composed of beliefs and desires (viz. Davidson, 1980). Hence in our example, the person comes to believe that the other person is in an anxious state, and desires or wants to do something to relieve this. Such an act can reasonably be characterised as an intentional act: it stems from beliefs and desires held by the actor, and aims at an outcome which the actor deliberately intends to bring about.

With reference to persons, a person described as caring, it is reasonable to suppose, can be relied upon to perform caring acts. For the description of the person as caring to be accurate, it would be expected that the person typically performs such acts.

And with reference to caring professions, it can be anticipated that these are professions which are associated with the undertaking of caring actions by their members. So to describe the medical profession as a caring profession would be to claim that the members of this profession are typically involved in the performance of caring acts.

Nothing has been said so far on the question of what it is that makes an act a caring act as opposed to some other type of act, for example a cruel act, but the observations just made suggest three features of them. First, that caring acts are intentional (that is, in the sense that they are deliberately undertaken and so on); the example of the giving of reassurance can be taken to suggest this. Second, caring acts are relational; that is, they are directed towards parties other than the actor – again, as in the 'reassurance' example just given. Third, and importantly, our discussion so far suggests that caring acts are directed towards meeting the needs or interests of others; in short, that caring acts are needs-related, where the needs in question are those of the party on the receiving end of the acts. Once more, this feature of caring acts is displayed in the 'reassurance' example.

It should be stressed that none of these three features is entirely unproblematic. For example, it has seemed plausible to some theorists to claim that caring is 'habitual', something closer to a reflex rather than a deliberate, consciously undertaken action (see, for example, Noddings, 1984, p. 3); so the suggestion that caring actions are necessarily intentional can be contended. (Although, nonetheless, such acts do seem to issue from beliefs and desires on the part of the actor; for example, a belief that a person is distressed and a desire to help her.) With regard to the view that caring is relational, one might contend this by advancing the claim that one can care for oneself. And lastly, with regard to the claim that caring acts are necessarily needs-related, one might point to an example such as caring for coin collection, or a vase, or any inanimate object. Here, it may be said a person performs caring actions which are not in any clear sense directed at the needs of the vase/coin collection.

In addition to the three features of caring actions just identified, we might note two 'poles' or extremes in the way the term 'care' is ordinarily used. At one end is a weak sense of the term which implies little, if any emotional involvement with what is cared for. At the other end is a very strong sense which does imply a very significant level of involvement with what is cared for.

As an example of the weaker sense consider polishing a vase or cleaning a car. Such an act is intentional, in the sense that it is deliberately carried out by the person doing the polishing; it stems from beliefs and desires (for example the belief that the car is dirty and the desire to have a clean car). The act is also relational in that it is directed at something other than the polisher. Is the act also needs-related? One might point to a sense in which it is. It is common to claim that a car or even a vase 'needs' cleaning or polishing.

However, even if it is allowed that ordinary usage is legitimate here, one can distinguish meeting these kinds of needs of inanimate things such as cars and vases from meeting the needs of humans in the following way. In the example given above of giving reassurance to someone, the point of this depends upon the fact of human vulnerability. Humans are beings with the capacity to suffer, to feel pain or pleasure. In philosophical terms, human experience has a phenomenology; there is something that it is like to be a human. This cannot properly be said of a car or a vase, and makes for a crucial difference in caring for humans in contrast to caring for inanimate objects.

So it has been suggested here that caring acts are intentional, are relational, and are needs-related. As noted, these features of caring acts apply equally to caring for inanimate objects as they do to caring for human beings. But due to obvious and important differences between humans and inanimate objects caring acts have a dimension in the context of human care that is necessarily lacking in the context of care for inanimate objects. Humans have a phenomenology, they can experience the world, they can suffer, there is something that it is like to be them; none of this is true of inanimate objects.

Hence the view that caring acts involve responses to needs can be retained. In the context of caring for humans, this requires on the part of the carer, appreciation of the facts of human vulnerability, their capacity to suffer and to experience the world. Caring for mere objects requires no such appreciation on the part of the carer. Thus we have identified a key difference in the mental attitude appropriately involved in the care of humans and inanimate objects: the former requires a conception of the cared for as essentially vulnerable, as a subject of experiences such as suffering and pleasure; the latter does not.

In the nursing context the sense of care identified here, that based upon the appreciation of the vulnerability of human beings, on their capacity for experiences such as suffering, is that which is minimally necessary for the nursing context. Any plausible account of caring within the nursing context must be one which recognises this aspect of the range of caring acts central to nursing; namely that they are directed at beings which have the capacity to experience pain, suffering or pleasure and which are recognised to have such a capacity. Appreciation of this feature of humans – their vulnerability – seems necessary for even the *intelligibility* of health care work. Such work, in nursing and medicine, seems logically posterior to the recognition of human suffering. It is the point, or *raison d'être* of these professions to provide a response to such suffering. It follows from this that the kinds of caring acts which are necessary to nursing are those which derive from a recognition that patients have the capacity to feel pain, and to suffer. Given this, it follows further, that the kind of caring appropriate to inanimate objects, is not appropriate to the nursing context. For the kind of caring appropriate to inanimate objects involves no presupposition of their possessing the capacity to suffer.

This conceptual truth about nursing (that is, necessary truth) is grounded in an inescapable feature of human existence such that humans are essentially vulnerable (they have the capacity to experience pain and suffering). Nursing can be understood as a moral response to this. Thus nursing is exposed as an essentially moral enterprise.

So the view that caring acts are responses to needs is being put forward here; and further, it is being claimed that recognition of the presence of needs in other humans requires a conception of others as beings with the capacity to suffer (and so on). The intelligibility of the nursing enterprise seems to rest upon this basic premise.

In addition to the appreciation of the fact of human vulnerability, it can be pointed out that humans have a point of view or perspective from which they experience the world. No two of us occupy exactly the same perspective. Since intentional caring in nursing requires consideration of the needs of the patient, it also plausibly requires consideration of what we previously termed the *plight* of the patient. This signals the morally salient features of the patient's situation. Thus it includes the phenomenological aspects of the patient's situation, and the more obviously narratival ones – the threat posed to the person's self-project by his illness, and the relationship between his symptoms and his past and present, and so on. It also signals the fact that illness does not simply involve disruption of parts of the body but disruption to the person.

The significance of trying to grasp this should be evident from our previous discussion of the importance of narrative understanding of patients. The patient's own view of his plight will have an important bearing upon what his needs are, and hence on what caring acts may be appropriate. But the idea of a plight makes room for the point that there is a perspective other than the patient's on his predicament. And this also is an important perspective in terms of the patient's nursing care.

So far then, we have noted that caring acts are intentional, relational and needs-related. In recognition of a distinction between caring for inanimate objects and caring for people, it was suggested that the latter requires a conception by the carer of the cared for as essentially vulnerable. This appears a plausible necessary condition of intentional caring within the nursing context. And, it marks both the moral nature of nursing, and the central place of intentional care within it.

We noted earlier a 'spectrum' of uses of the term care. One view of caring which appears very strong indeed is described in the following passage from Watson:

> Caring is viewed as the moral ideal of nursing where there is utmost concern for human dignity and preservation of humanity. Human care can begin when the nurse enters into the life space or phenomenal field of another person, is able to detect the other person's condition of being (spirit, soul), feels this condition within him or herself and responds to the condition in such a way that the recipient has a release of subjective feelings and thoughts he or she had been longing to release...
> (Watson, quoted in van Hooft, 1987, p. 29; see also Watson, 1988, p. 31).

This description of what is involved in caring within nursing goes much further than the minimal requirement identified above. On the minimal view, what is required is appreciation of the vulnerability of the patient, and response to this. Consider how this differs from the view expressed here by Watson. In her view, caring requires the nurse to experience the patient's predicament as this is experienced by the patient. For her, when the nurse does this it has a cathartic effect upon the patient, in that it causes a 'release' of pent-up emotions.

Caring in this sense appears very demanding indeed. It requires almost complete immersion in the perspective of the patient, 'feeling' the patient's condition within himself, and giving each patient 'utmost concern'. In fact, this characterisation of caring does not seem a very plausible requirement within the nursing context. As van Hooft indicates (1987), there seem serious practical obstacles to the implementation of such a view of caring: for example in terms of the time required developing such close relationships with patients. Also, again as van Hooft suggests, such a level of involvement may be wholly inappropriate. Patients might reasonably wish to refrain from any involvement with a nurse in a relationship of the intensity described by Watson.

Moreover, there are obvious problems in the requirement to 'feel' another's predicament as they themselves feel it; suppose the patient is in agony. And it is not ontologically possible: one cannot experience a person's pain in the way they themselves do. Watson's requirement of a cathartic response by the patient seems inappropriate too. A caring act *may* have the kind of effect Watson requires, for example giving an anxious patient reassurance might do so. But it seems clear that such acts *need not* have such an effect, for example holding a patient's hand out of concern for their health, gently bathing a patient, feeding a patient, each seem legitimately described as caring acts, but they need not have the cathartic outcome Watson requires. So the view of caring, as represented in the passage from Watson quoted, is a stronger one than that so far set out here, but it does not seem a plausible one: it is excessively strong.

It can be observed, then, that discussions of intentional care within nursing have a fairly tricky path to negotiate. They must avoid being so weak as to allow the kinds of caring acts appropriate to caring for inanimate objects. But they must also avoid being excessively demanding, so they become either professionally inappropriate, ontologically impossible, or practically implausible. The sketch presented here so far is one which permits a distinction between the kinds of caring acts appropriate to human patients and to inanimate objects. It is grounded in an ontological distinction between them, and in the necessity of recognition of this (if only tacitly) in caring acts upon them. Also, it is grounded in a crucial difference in the kinds of needs which inanimate objects can intelligibly be claimed to possess, and the kinds of needs which human patients can intelligibly be said to possess. Humans have needs which are rooted in their essential vulnerability. Humans have a point of view on the world, and can experience it. These notions have no application to inanimate objects.

We turn now to discuss some aspects of the pioneering work on the topic of care undertaken by Noddings. The discussion will provide an opportunity to try to cement further the sketch of intentional care provided so far, and to note some difficulties with Noddings' own line. It should be said in advance that a difficulty to be faced by Noddings' account of care also faces the sketch presented so far here, this concerns the nursing care of humans in persistent vegetative states (PVS).

Noddings and care

Noddings (1984) is a theorist who has provided a detailed account of caring which is widely respected and referred to in nursing literature. Fry, for example, writes 'Noddings' model [of caring] is a rich ground for the future discussion of nursing ethics' (Fry, 1989, p. 9; also Bishop and Scudder, 1991, pp. 67–76). In accordance with what was said above, Noddings proposes that care is a relational concept (1984, p. 19). In order for it to be the case that a person cares there has to be a thing or person cared for; thus caring is importantly 'other-regarding'.

With regard to the attitude of caring itself on the part of the person caring, Noddings proposes that this involves a 'displacement of interest from my own reality to the reality of the other' (ibid., p. 14). Caring for another, she proposes, involves: 'Apprehending the other's reality, feeling what he feels as nearly as possible, [this] is the essential part of caring from the view of the one-caring' (ibid., p. 16). And:

> Caring involves stepping out of one's own personal frame of reference into the other's. When we care, we consider the other's point of view, [and]... his objective needs (1984, p. 24).

So the general focus of Noddings' view also lies on the attempt to grasp what we earlier termed the plight of the person being cared for. As with Watson, there is a danger here that Noddings requires that which is ontologically impossible: that is, 'stepping out of one's own frame of reference'. This is dubious on the grounds that it is simply not possible to step out of one's own frame of reference. One views the world through a set of concepts and values, for example the concepts of a person, of pain and suffering, and innumerable others. These cannot simply be jettisoned.

Perhaps Noddings' point is a weaker one, namely that captured in the final quoted sentence – that is, that 'we consider the other's point of view'. Providing we note that this can only be done through the lens of our own 'frame of reference', this is unobjectionable and, indeed, coheres with what was proposed earlier concerning the importance of considering the plight of the person being cared for.

On this weaker view, then, from the perspective of the carer, caring necessarily involves appreciating the position of the cared-for 'as nearly as possible' 1984, p. 24). And considering and respecting the 'objective needs' of the cared-for – although again, presumably, one could only do this 'as far as possible' (ibid., p. 24). Note that this marks a clear contrast with the view put forward by Watson; for her, one is required to experience what the person being cared for experiences as he himself experiences it. But for Noddings, at least when interpreted in the weaker way just described, in caring for persons, one is required only to appreciate how the person is feeling, and then respond to his needs. (It should be added, however, that Noddings can be read in the 'strong' way also, such that caring requires a strong level of involvement with the person cared for – 'engrossment' (ibid., p. 33), as she puts it.)

Minimally, then, caring involves the appreciation of the perspective of the person being cared for. When one has done this, one is in a position to determine that person's needs, and to try to respond to them. There are likely to be situations in which this strategy proves extremely difficult to implement, for example in caring for a person from a culture radically different from one's own. But if communication is possible with such a person, there is at least that avenue to make use of to try to determine how things are for that person; one can simply ask them how they are feeling, what they would like, and so on. It is worth noting Noddings' recognition of the fact that one cannot simply occupy the perspective of another, one can only do so 'as far as possible'. But this aspect of caring, considering the perspective of the person being cared for, is plainly a crucial element of intentional care.

Thus two features of Noddings' view (in its weaker version) can be supported here:

1. Caring involves appreciation of the plight of another, where this requires some conception of the person's own view of his plight on the part of the carer, and

2. Caring acts require responding, on the basis of this 'appreciation'; typically this will take the form of trying to meet some discerned need or needs of the person being cared for.

Care as reciprocal

We turn now to a more controversial aspect of Noddings' thesis. We noted earlier her recognition of care as relational, but Noddings goes much further than merely to note the relational component of care. Interestingly, she proposes that for it to be true that one person A cares for another person B, then B 'must contribute appropriately' (1984, p. 19); that is, the relationship must be 'completed' in some way by B. The nature of this contribution involves receiving the care (1984, p. 69). Examples of what Noddings has in mind by this receiving indicate that the person cared for responds in such a way that it is possible for the carer to engage with the cared-for. Noddings writes:

> A mother describes her two babies and the difference in responsiveness to her. As she holds one on her knee, the child looks right at her, responding to her smiles, frowns and funny faces. The other child, held in the same playful attitude, looks across the room. Both children are very bright and pleasant, but the mother confesses that she enjoys her responsive baby more. He is fun to be with. She is a bit baffled by the other (1984, p. 71).

Here, then, the kind of responsiveness which the first baby displays, for Noddings, makes the 'completion' of the caring relationship possible. Where there is no such responsiveness, controversially, she claims such completion is not possible. One might reasonably suppose it could be the case that one person cares for another in the absence of there being any reciprocity of feeling between them.

The reason is that regardless of whether the person being cared for responds, one might still perform the kind of intentional act that is required in caring for a person. If intentional caring requires a recognition on the part of the carer of the vulnerability of the other person, and of his needs, then it seems possible to perform a caring act in relation to that person. But Noddings' account requires more than this. Specifically, that the care is reciprocated in some way. But surely this is mistaken. For example, suppose a patient is compulsorily detained in hospital under the *Mental Health Act* (1983). Such a patient may be extremely hostile to nursing staff because of this. But a nurse might still be able to care for that person by considering the perspective of that person in the way Noddings describes, and by trying to determine and respond to that patient's needs.

Consider also the difficulties involved in caring for people with conditions such as autism. In severe cases of this disorder autistic people shun contact with others and seem not to 'return' any care shown to them. But surely, a parent of such an autistic child could care for the child. So I would suggest that Noddings' reciprocity requirement is too strong and should not be included among the necessary constituents of acts of intentional caring.

We turn now to a second controversial aspect of Noddings's position on the topic of care. This concerns the 'origin' of what she terms 'ethical caring'; that is, for present purposes, intentional caring of the kind with which we are concerned to explicate here.

Why care?

Noddings suggests that we recognise the moral significance of caring as a result of recollections of our own experiences of being cared for – specifically in the mother–child relationship (1984, p. 79) – and this she terms 'natural caring'. As she puts it: 'Ethical caring' arises out of our experiences of 'natural caring' (ibid.). The distinction here is supposed to acknowledge that we would not standardly describe a mother's caring for her baby as an example of a moral act. It is a caring act, but one which does not stem from recognition of any kind of obligation; it is 'instinctive', natural. Hence caring of this type can be termed natural caring. Ethical caring is prompted by the recognition of the needs of another, for example generated by the suffering of another. Recognition of their suffering produces a 'call' in us, or put in other terms, a 'moral pull'. If we opt to answer that call, our actions are characterised as ethical caring in Noddings' view.

Thus Noddings writes:

> The source of ethical behaviour is, then, in twin sentiments – one that feels directly for the other and one that feels for and with that best self, who may accept and sustain the initial feeling rather than reject it (1984, p. 80).

So on this account we have an initial 'feeling' for another person, in the case of a person who is clearly suffering, their plight calls out to us, or exerts a moral pull on us. If we respond to this call or pull, our acts are acts of ethical caring. Such acts are those of our 'best self', that person we strive to be, a morally virtuous person. Hence, in accordance with the directions of our 'best self' we respond to the 'feeling for the other'.

Noddings' proposal that ethical caring arises out of natural caring is a very strong and controversial one. It amounts to the view that it is necessary to have experienced natural caring in order to be capable of ethical caring. But of course it seems plausible to suppose that a person who has not experienced such natural caring may well still prove capable of ethical caring. It is reasonable to suppose a person could come to appreciate the fact of human vulnerability, and human need in spite of not having experienced natural caring. Indeed, such deprivation may heighten a person's sensitivity to these dimensions of human experience and motivate them to care for others.

So, as with the requirement of reciprocity in the caring relation, the proposal that the experience of natural caring is a necessary condition of the capacity for ethical caring does not seem plausible. It seems easy to conceive that a person may have been brought up in circumstances such that he is deprived of any experience of natural caring, but that such a person becomes extremely morally sensitive, becomes a good, caring person. So the experience of natural caring does not seem a likely necessary condition for ethical caring. Nor does it seem a plausible sufficient condition. A person may be raised by caring parents, and thus experience natural caring, and yet still turn out to be evil or morally abhorrent.

Finally, the fact that Noddings' discussion of care takes place within the framework of moral philosophy should not be lost sight of. The claim that caring acts have a moral dimension, deriving in part from the view that they are responses to the vulnerability of others is an important one; in such an account, as we heard, caring acts answer a moral call, or 'pull'. If this is so, we can claim that acts of intentional caring have a moral dimension. This derives in part from the attitude of the carer, but also from the fact that such acts, as we have described them here, 'aim at' a good – this being either the relief of suffering, the promoting of well-being, or the meeting of the (legitimate) needs of another.

In summary, Noddings' line, when shorn of 'reciprocity' and 'natural caring' requirements, coheres with the sketch of intentional caring advanced earlier. Her view allows us to distinguish caring for inanimate objects from caring about persons. Since one cannot, in any interesting sense, consider the perspective of an inanimate object one cannot care about that object in the same way in which one can care about a person. One can care about a person since a person is a subject of experience: there is something that it is like to *be* that person. One can imagine what kinds of beliefs and desires the person may be entertaining, and one can imagine what kinds of experiences the person is undergoing. Hence, it is intelligible to consider how the world seems from the perspective of that person. It is not plausible to say that inanimate objects are the subjects of experience and that one can care about them in the same way in which one can care about persons. Similarly, from the perspective of needs, one can articulate clear and significant differences between the kinds of acts appropriate in caring for persons, and acts appropriate to caring for inanimate objects.

Care, emotion and two problems

A further interesting dimension to discussions of intentional care in recent years has focused on the role of emotion in caring (see for example, Nortvedt, 1996, 1998; Scott, 2000). The idea is that there is a close connection between emotion and caring seems very plausible. So we now turn to a brief consideration of that line with the ultimate aim of clarifying a sense of intentional care which is *central to*, if not *exclusive to*, nursing.

As we noted, a plausible necessary condition of caring involves attempting to grasp the perspective of the person being cared for, for example their vulnerability. The view of that perspective as exerting a 'moral pull' on the carer is claimed by Nortvedt (1998) to involve 'emotional understanding' (p. 387) on the part of the carer. Put simply, being affected by another, feeling sorrow, anguish, anger, disgust or joy involves an emotional understanding of the other's plight. The contrast here is between a purely cognitive recognition of the other's plight, and a recognition which, since imbued with emotional understanding, exerts a moral pull on us.

For Nortvedt (1996, 1998) the presence of an emotional element in each caring act is a necessary, inescapable feature of such acts. One way to make this claim sound plausible is to 'build in' the idea of emotional sensitivity into the grasping of another's plight. Since caring requires the latter, it would then follow that caring requires the former.

In appraising such a claim it can be observed that there do seem clear cases in which emotion is involved in nursing practice: for example, assisting at a birth, nursing a patient who is suffering greatly, and so on. In situations of these types the place of emotion and emotional understanding seems plain. But there also seem situations which involve caring but do not, at least obviously, involve emotion. For example, giving a patient a routine oral medication, casually speaking to a patient, or, removing a ball-bearing which has become lodged in a person's ear. In cases such as these awareness of the plight of the patient remains necessary, but emotion seems not to be involved.

However, it can be argued that the very process of leading our lives, dealing with the events, in our actions and decisions, inescapably involves emotion at some level. So *all* acts, not simply those which are acts of intentional caring, stem from emotional sensitivity at some level (see Heidegger, 1962, p. 175; Taylor, 1985; van Hooft, 1995). Roughly speaking, such a claim is advanced on the grounds that our acts reveal what matters to us: running from an attacker, rushing to help an accident victim, or more mundanely, making tea, getting dressed. These acts have an affective dimension at some level in the sense that they reveal what we care about, what we value (see, for example, Heidegger, 1962; van Hooft, 1995, p. 55).

This is a view which can be exploited by a proponent of the claim that all caring acts involve an emotional component. This allows us to distinguish two accounts of what is occurring in intentional caring actions in nursing. In the first account, the caring act is a response to the patient on the basis of a perceived need of the patient; this requires some capacity to conceive of the plight of the patient on the part of the nurse. Perhaps sympathy will serve as an indication of the kind of mental act which is involved here (this issue will be returned to in Chapter 7). In this first view, caring acts *may* have an emotional element – for example in the extreme cases of suffering noted earlier. But on this first view an act can be a caring act without *necessarily* having an emotional element. So on this first view an emotional component is not a necessary, but a contingent feature of caring acts. Thus, on this first view, it is only contingently true of caring acts that they have an emotional component. It is not necessarily true that they have such a component.

A second view, one held by Nortvedt, holds that an emotional element *is* a necessary component of a caring act. The reason is that, in this account, appreciation of the plight of another necessarily involves emotional sensitivity. So the presence of an emotional element is a necessary and not a mere contingent feature of caring acts.

So, we noted a claim to the effect that intentional care requires 'emotional understanding' on the part of the carer. This opened up the possibility of identifying a necessary feature of caring acts, via the inclusion of an emotional component. However, against this it was pointed out that many perfectly proper nursing acts seem not to have an emotional element to them, for example acts involving care of a 'routine' nature.

However, in favour of the view that all caring acts have an emotional component we can recruit some of the claims of Heidegger. In his view, it seems that 'mood' is a central, inescapable feature of leading a human life. In other words that, in leading our lives, we inescapably have a 'mood', some mood or other (Heidegger, 1962, p. 173). Thus it is said that our lives have an emotional 'tone', whether one feels flat, or excited, or angry, or fearful, or bored, or some other. If this is correct, and it does sound a plausible claim, all acts, not simply those of intentional caring will include an emotional component. This follows since, if the Heideggerian line is accepted, all our acts take place within the context of our enduring some 'mood' or other. As noted, this can be read as signifying that we lead our lives in some emotional register. In support of the Heideggerian claim concerning the ever-present nature of mood, a remark of van Hooft's is instructive here. He points out 'The world is not neutral to our gaze' (1995, p. 55); we view the world in terms of its significance to us at some level. And it seems reasonable to anchor the idea of significance in affective terms. Thus, since it turns out that all our actions now have an emotional element to them, it follows of course that so too do caring acts.

It is necessary now to draw attention to two possible problems with the account of intentional caring sketched here so far. The first concerns the possibility of caring for humans in PVS; the second concerns beings such as non-human animals which lie 'between', so to speak, humans and inanimate objects.

The problem of humans in PVS

Humans in persistent vegetative states constitute a problem for any account of intentional caring which requires consideration of the perspective of the cared for. From a purely phenomenological perspective, such beings do not differ from inanimate objects. (Of course this problem must be faced by Noddings' account of care also.)

Perhaps it is enough in these troubling and tragic cases that they have a history of having such a perspective, and a history of phenomenological experience. Also, they are typically involved in relations with others in a way in which inanimate objects are not. A point such as this, perhaps in conjunction with the fact of the relatedness within social networks of these individuals may be recruited here. These kinds of observations do enough to suggest that the moral status of such individuals is not simply that of inanimate objects – as noted, their social relations, human form, and phenomenological history help to resist such a conclusion.

Moreover, as noted previously it is reported that nurses caring for humans in PVS actually construct perspectives for them, describing their own social lives, interacting with the patient as if the patient still possessed the capacity for a 'perspective' (de Raeve, 1996).

Perhaps the idea of a plight can do some work here as suggested earlier (Chapter 5). For although shorn of a self-project, and of the phenomenological aspects of human experience, such patients can still be said to have a plight, a tragic one. And this can be invoked to help to explain, if only partially, why it remains possible to intentionally care for such patients.

Lastly, what of Noddings' claim that caring involves protecting interests and 'objective needs' (1984, p. 24), could this be recruited to uphold the idea of intentional caring in this context? This does not seem a promising strategy to me. For of course the idea of interests seems most plausibly bound to beings which can experience pleasure or pain, or flourish in some sense. This does not apply to humans in PVS. And the appeal to 'objective needs' is vulnerable to objection on the grounds that, say, a car might have such needs, for example for servicing (that is, unless it is serviced it will cease to function).

So the best one can do to salvage the idea of intentional caring as it applies to humans in PVS is to emphasise that the difficulty in applying that notion to 'care' of such people, does nothing to impugn their moral standing. Also, the relatives of such people will clearly be in need of intentional care. And lastly, perhaps paradoxically such cases really strengthen the sketch of intentional care put forward here since those nurses caring for such people appear to 'construct' a narrative for them in terms of their self-project prior to being in PVS.

Caring for non-human animals

Problematically, non-human animals, notably pets, feature 'between', so to speak, humans and inanimate objects, and it might be claimed that it is possible to intentionally care for them. It is reasonable to suppose they too are vulnerable, have a phenomenology, a perspective on the world and a plight.

Two responses to this observation seem possible. The first sees no difficulty in generalising across to such animals the idea of intentional caring. Those sympathetic to this strategy will presumably see no problem here. However, others may not be content with this and hold out for the view that intentional caring has a legitimate application in the care of humans only. Proponents of this view might take a second strategy. They may point out that, as sketched here, intentional caring requires a grasp of the plight of the cared for. It may then be pointed out that, as humans, we have so little a conception of what it is like to be a dog or a cat, still less a snake or other kind of reptile that the language of intentional caring has no proper application in such contexts.

Having noted these two responses, I would suggest that there is no need to get involved in that further debate here since our main concern lies within the nursing context (see, for example, Singer, 1990).

Lastly, it is worth stressing once more that on the sketch advanced here one can easily appreciate that groups other than nurses care: parents can be said to care about their offspring, social workers may care about their clients, and so on.

Conclusion

It has been claimed that a plausible account of acts of intentional caring within the nursing context must be one which requires they are directed at vulnerable beings which have a plight, standardly, this includes a phenomenology. Appreciation of such features of humans seems necessary for even the intelligibility of health care work. Caring acts stem from a conception of the plight of the patient, and will be needs-related.

Thus noting an ontological feature of human existence (vulnerability: the capacity to experience pain and suffering) enables us to observe that the intelligibility of nursing rests upon this feature. Nursing can, hence, be understood as a moral response to human vulnerability, pain and suffering, and thus to involve, inevitably, acts of intentional care.

This kind of caring will differ from the kind described by Watson above for reasons given earlier. The kind of care described here also differs from the very weak kind of care involved in caring for inanimate objects. Since such objects have no perspective, plight or phenomenology, they cannot be objects of nursing care.

The account of care suggested here entails that caring will not be unique to nursing. However this should be regarded as a strength and not a weakness. It is implausible to suppose that there is a kind of caring unique to nursing.

The claim has been made here that acts of intentional caring within the nursing context are acts which require, as a necessary condition, a conception of the plight of the patient, in standard cases, as an individual with the capacity to suffer.

The relationship between caring actions and emotion has also been discussed briefly. Two views were identified: in the first, caring acts need not necessarily have an emotional element, in the second, they do. It was argued that all acts have such a component since it is a feature of human being – leading a human life – that things, inescapably, matter to one. This 'mattering' signals an emotional dimension to human existence.

Finally, then, according to the sketch presented so far, acts of intentional care require:

1. a conception of the plight of the cared for
2. a response to their needs
3. an emotional component

It has also been maintained that caring acts have a moral dimension: not least in the sense that they stem from a response to the 'moral pull' exerted by a conception of the plight of another; thus caring acts may be prompted by caring.

7 Care in nursing (ii): ontological care

Having discussed the idea of intentional care in Chapter 6, our focus now is on the idea of ontological care; that is, on the idea of care as an inescapable feature of leading a human life. As we will see, this ontological sense of care is divisible into two kinds: 'deep' care, and 'identity constituting' care. Deep care concerns the basic, biological level of human existence. Identity constituting care concerns the sense in which what we care about makes us the person we are. Our discussion concludes with an outline of how the idea of ontological care relates to that of intentional care. It will be shown that a nurse is better equipped to provide intentional care, if he has an understanding of the idea of ontological care.

Ontological care

We noted at the beginning of Chapter 6 a distinction between intentional and ontological care. Acts of intentional caring were said to be kinds of actions which stem from deliberate, intentional actions on the part of human carers. The topic of ontological care is to be discussed in this section. This is a form of care which is claimed to be a necessary feature of all humans. Thus Benner and Wrubel claim caring is part of what it is to be a human being. As they put it 'Caring is a basic way of being in the world' (1989, p. xi; p. 368), and they describe nursing as 'a caring practice' (ibid.), hence the title of their book *The Primacy of Caring*.

In contrast with intentional care, ontological 'care' is considered by Benner and Wrubel to derive from a level of care which is rooted in the 'being' of humans in a much deeper way than mere intentional care. Care in this sense is so deeply rooted that it can be severed from the 'intentional realm', from the realm of conscious thought. It is claimed that one can 'care' in a sense to be made clear, without having consciously decided to care. (Though as we will see later, one type of ontological care will turn out to be related to the 'intentional realm'.)

The reason is that care, it is held, is an essential, inescapable part of the make-up of human beings. So when Benner and Wrubel claim that 'Caring is a basic way of being in the world' (1989, p. xi) they should be taken as claiming that it is part of the very nature of humans, so to speak, to care. Recalling, of course, that the kind of care under discussion *need not* be intentional. According to their claim, it is a necessary truth about humans that humans care.

Given this view of care – as a feature which is part of the very make-up and constitution of humans – we can describe it as an ontological view. For as we heard in Chapter 1, ontology involves the enquiry into the very natures of things, into the characteristics which are necessarily true of them. Hence the claim that care is so fundamental to being human is an ontological claim.

Thus ontological caring is a form of caring which is part of 'human being', part of what it is to lead a human life, and to be human. This appeal to caring as a way of being in the world is derived from the work of Heidegger (1962), as Benner and Wrubel acknowledge. For example, Heidegger writes: 'Dasein, when understood ontologically is care [*sorge*]' (1962, p. 84, p. 237, part V, *passim*).

In crude elaboration of this very difficult and complex claim, Heidegger can be interpreted as follows. 'Dasein' is Heidegger's term for human persons, and can be understood literally as 'being there'. What he is pointing to is that as humans we inevitably find ourselves in the midst of things, we are 'thrown' into the world. As a result of this we have no option other than to do our best to deal with, or cope with, the situation we find ourselves in.

Heidegger's view, is usefully described as follows:

> Dasein is always occupied with the entities it encounters in the world... The point is not that Dasein is always caring and concerned, or that failures of sympathy are impossible or to be discouraged; it is rather that, as Being-in-the-world, Dasein must deal with that world. The world and everything in it is something that cannot fail to matter to it (Mulhall, 1996, p. 111).

This passage draws attention to two crucial aspects of Heidegger's claims about care, one negative and one positive. First, the negative point can be stated very briefly. This is that care in Heidegger's sense is not synonymous with intentional care, hence the claim 'The point is not that Dasein is always caring and concerned...' (ibid.). So for Heidegger, and thus also for Benner and Wrubel, 'care' in the ontological sense is not care in the intentional sense. It is not the kind of care one might appeal to in saying of a kind act 'That was a caring thing to do'.

Second, more positively, Heidegger's view is that by virtue of our inevitably being situated within the world – being surrounded by people, objects, by our having needs, feelings and desires – we are compelled to 'deal' with the world, with the situations within which we find ourselves. Hence, it is in this sense that the world inevitably matters to us. But this 'mattering' need not be the result of conscious deliberation on our part. Within situations we make choices, some reflective, some less so. Thus our actions reveal what matters to us, whether or not these acts result from conscious, reflective choices.

One way to explicate this idea is by consideration of human being – of what it is to lead a human life. Consider the basic, biological aspect of such 'being' (that is, of living). From the moment of birth (and even prior to this), we have to deal with the world. The biological element of our nature ensures that needs for oxygen, water, food and comfort make themselves known to us if they are not met. This aspect of our being never leaves us. At what we might term the 'social level' of human being, similarly, the world cannot fail to matter to us. It impresses itself upon us inescapably. In interacting with others we have to interpret their words, their body language, posture and moods. If we retreat into solitude the urge for company inevitably arises. We have to choose whether to answer it or suppress it.

It is this feature of what it is to be a human being – in Heidegger's terms, of human Being-in-the-world – that Heidegger describes by the term care (*sorge*). Thus, recall the enigmatic quote given above, 'Dasein, when understood ontologically is care' (1962, p. 84). It is an inescapable part of what it is to be human that humans are situated, and that, inevitably things matter to them. Ontologically speaking, this is what it is, for Heidegger, to propose that Dasein's being is care.

So ontological care in Heidegger's sense, is part of the very nature of humans. And, to stress this point, it certainly should not be read as a claim to the effect that all humans are 'caring' people, concerned for the welfare and well-being of others. This would be a deeply implausible claim, and it is not one which can be found within Heidegger, and it must be supposed, it is not one advanced by Benner and Wrubel.

However, as noted earlier, the idea of ontological caring as central to nursing has been brought to prominence by Benner and Wrubel (1989). But of course, the account of care provided by Heidegger applies to all humans, and not simply to nurses; his is an account of human being, not simply of what it is to be a nurse.

A worry then is this: if the idea of ontological caring applies to all humans, in what sense is it relevant to nursing? The enquiries into caring either attempted by nurse theorists, or recruited by them are typically for the purpose of articulating a mode of caring either central to nursing, or even unique to nursing (Leininger, 1984; Watson, 1988; Benner and Wrubel, 1989). But the turn toward ontological caring, on examination, may not advance the project of articulating a form of caring central to nursing. All that project uncovers in the work of Heidegger is a dimension of human being common to all humans. So, does this entail that the turn to ontological caring is ultimately a dead-end? I will try to show that it is not, but for reasons which, I suspect, differ from those usually taken to be the case.

Before doing this, we return to consider again Benner and Wrubel's claims for the primacy of caring within nursing.

Benner and Wrubel's appeal to ontological caring

Benner and Wrubel write:

> Caring as it is used in this book means that persons, events, projects, and things matter to people. Caring is essential if the person is to live in a differentiated world where some things really matter, while others are less important or not important at all... [The] term caring is used appropriately to describe a wide range of involvements, from romantic love to parental love to friendship, from caring for one's garden to caring about one's work to caring for and about one's patients.
>
> Caring sets up the condition that something or someone outside the person matters and creates personal concerns. Without care, the person would be without projects and concerns. Care sets up a world and creates meaningful distinctions... (1989, p. 1).

The concept of care appealed to here is required to do a great deal of work. In this passage, they use 'care' in both intentional and ontological senses. The second sentence indicates that care is prior to the identification of concerns or intentional cares, and this is echoed in the final sentence also – that is, 'Care sets up a world...'. Thus these sentences seem tacitly to refer to the ontological sense of care. Crudely, care at the ontological level, as so far described, 'sets up a world' in the sense that the way we lead our lives inescapably reflects, for example, the biological aspect of our being, described earlier. So at a basic level, our biology entails that certain things must matter to us; most primitively these include basic biological needs. So a world is set up for us, in the sense that its organisation cannot be in ignorance of our biological dimension. (See also van Hooft (1995) on ontological care.)

With regard to intentional caring, it is in the third sentence as quoted above that this seems most prominent, hence the reference to caring for persons, patients and so on. It should be said that the tacit reference to intentional care here appears to ignore what seems an important distinction, one we discussed in the previous section, between caring for humans, and for inanimate objects.

Hence it is plain that, without warning the reader, Benner and Wrubel appeal to a highly technical sense of 'care' which, as they make plain, they are recruiting from the work of Heidegger (1962). In lumping together all these importantly different senses of care, at best, they seem open to the charge of invoking a highly technical term without warning the reader of it. More critically, they may be charged with encouraging an unwarranted conflation of ontological and intentional care, thus misleading any readers who are unaware of these subtleties.

Two senses of ontological care: deep care and identity-constituting care

In order to try to make clear what I take to be important in Benner and Wrubel's discussion of care, it will be necessary to distinguish two types of care within the category of ontological care.

The first sense we can term 'deep care' (I borrow this expression from van Hooft, 1995, p. 29). This sense of care is furthest removed from the intentional realm (the realm of conscious thought). It is this sense which is best exemplified by reference to the biological level of human being. Thus, an unconscious person still retains this caring aspect to her being, although of course she could not act intentionally and so could not perform an act of intentional caring (at least during the period in which she is unconscious).

The second sense is less easily separated from the intentional realm, although it remains ontological, and the term 'identity-constituting care' is used here to refer to it. This sense is captured summarily in the idea that *we are constituted by our cares*, so to speak. I take this to be another way of expressing the narrative view of the person described above in Chapter 5. Put in terms of 'care', we noted that a person's self-project is characterised by their values and goals. We can express this by stating that such self-projects manifest what people care about.

To explain this, suppose one is asked the question 'Who are you?' There is a clear sense in which merely giving one's name is not an answer to this question. In trying to answer it one is invited to describe what it is that one takes to be distinctive of one. Thus a person may say he is the father of two children, is a nurse, and originates from Birmingham. In relating these details, the person reveals just what it is they take to be important to their lives; put another way they reveal what they care about. So in giving a description of whom they are, a person's identity can be seen to be defined in terms of what they most care about. This will be evident also in the person's actions. Choosing to act in one way rather than another exposes what it is that one cares more about. Suppose, for example, that a person, when given the choice between doing academic work and spending time with his children chooses to do the former (outside of 'official' work time). If this is a pattern of behaviour, and if the person's continued employment does not require such a prioritising, it seems reasonable to suppose they attach very considerable weight to their academic work; they care about it greatly.

Developing this a little further, it can be said that the person conceives of themselves as a kind of person who places a high value on academic activity. This, it may be said, is a crucial part of their identity (or their self-interpretation as Benner and Wrubel put it (1989)).

As a further example, consider the professional footballer David Beckham. Reports suggest that from a very young age Beckham has wanted to be a professional footballer. It is plausible to suppose that if asked to say who he is, he would describe himself in such terms (in addition to others: a father, a husband, and so on). Of course there are many activities that Beckham engages in, such as tea drinking let us say. But it is very unlikely that he would cite this in answer to the kind of identity question we have been discussing. It is unlikely he would describe himself as a 'tea drinker', or that he would regard this to be as important in his life as playing football.

These points are intended to try to elaborate the view that we can be 'constituted by our cares'. They suggest that the individual identities of persons are expressed in terms of what matters most to them. And it should be stressed that we are not here articulating an account of persons which differs from the narrative account. Rather, we are expressing the same account in slightly different terms – invoking the sense of care uncovered in our investigation of ontological care.

Let us now apply some of these considerations to the nursing context. Suppose one becomes ill, and suppose that one cares a great deal about one's work. If the illness is even only moderately serious, it is likely that the extent to which one can enact such cares becomes restricted. Hence chronic illness can be predicted to have a devastating impact upon a person. For that person is likely to suppose he will not be able to pursue his cares, at least not in the way done hitherto. Chronic illness typically impacts upon most areas of a person's life, and thus, in terms of care, will impinge upon a person's capacity to pursue his cares; these might be family members, or work-projects, or political campaigns.

Alternatively take Beckham and the academic described briefly above. A knee injury to the academic may mean very little to him. For it has little impact upon his capacity to pursue his cares. This is not so for Beckham. Assuming he describes himself as a professional footballer, a knee injury has far more significance for him than for the academic. It may impugn his capacity to pursue his cares. More seriously, if he defines himself in terms of being a footballer he may perceive such an injury as a threat to his very identity. Such an injury has the potential to shatter his own conception of who he is.

Benner and Wrubel usefully point to the view that it is crucial for the nurse to grasp what it is that the patient is most concerned about in order for the nurse to act therapeutically. So in order to care for the patient, the nurse needs to determine just what the patient cares about. When the nurse grasps this, she will be better equipped to help him cope with the stress of his illness. It is important to note that what the nurse is required to appreciate is the patient's own interpretation of his predicament; that is, the patient's own view of the seriousness or otherwise of his symptoms. This is the case even if the patient's view differs markedly from the opinion of others. For it is the patient's interpretation of his situation which generates the patient's stress.

So in order for a nurse to perform acts of intentional care it will be necessary for the nurse to consider care at the ontological level: about what does the patient most care? how is she interpreting her symptoms in terms of their impact upon what she cares about? Thus it will be necessary to take into account care at the ontological level; specifically, it will be necessary to take into account identity-constituting care. Patients will interpret their symptoms in terms of their perceived impact upon their capacity to pursue what they care about. This may be work, hobbies, relations, or other family commitments. (Needless to add, vulnerability as an essential characteristic of human beings is a further ontological aspect of them which is central to nursing. As argued earlier, it is something upon which the very intelligibility of nursing rests.)

However, Benner and Wrubel's presentation of such a position requires clarification, of the kind undertaken here. Readers of Benner and Wrubel tend not to distinguish the senses of the term care described herein.

In summary then, as we have seen, ontological care is a feature of human beings in general. It is not unique to nurses, nor to patients. However, more positively, Benner and Wrubel bring out the importance of the fact that people have a conception of the situations within which they are embedded. Such conceptions may be sources of stress and anxiety. Given that a key role of the nurse is to help people cope with their illnesses, or symptoms, it seems important that nurses should try to appreciate or grasp patients' conceptions of their predicaments.

This seems to me to be the key point of the attempt to articulate the idea of 'ontological care'. But it seems fair to say that this is not widely recognised within nursing literature (but see Paley, 2000). For, due largely to confusion regarding the precise character of Benner and Wrubel's appeal to Heidegger and care, the difference between ontological and intentional care is simply not recognised. I suspect that most nurse readers of Benner and Wrubel expect to be informed of the kind of intentional attitude which characterises nurses' caring; rather, on a sympathetic reading at least, Benner and Wrubel do not do this. What they do is explain the importance of patients' conceptions of their predicaments. Such conceptions stem from ontological caring, from the view that 'Dasein, when understood ontologically is care' (Heidegger, 1962, p. 84).

In summary then, in spite of the emergence of appeals to ontological caring within nursing, this notion seems too general to contribute to the task of articulating a sense of 'care' which is unique to nursing. The reason, as we have seen, is that the ontological aspect of care applies to all humans and so will not help to mark out a sense of caring distinct to nursing. Nonetheless, as seen above, an appreciation of the idea of identity constituting care seems central to nursing. Obtaining a view of just what the patient cares about is crucial to the proper nursing care of patients.

Recap

Having now discussed intentional and ontological care, it is time to try to outline a view on how these might be related, with specific reference to the nursing context. Three types of care can now usefully be discerned. The first is the kind of deep ontological care exemplified by our discussion of the biological level of human being. This is separable from the intentional realm. The second is also a form of ontological care but this concerns the sense in which we are constituted by our cares – as just discussed; henceforth, we will term this 'identity-constituting care'. To repeat, this is an ontological claim since it is a claim about the constitution of persons by their cares, so to speak. The third type of care is intentional care. This is the kind of care with which we began our discussion; it is the kind of care with which discussions of care within nursing literature are typically concerned.

This threefold division, then, invokes a distinction between two types of ontological care: deep care and identity-constituting care. The third type of care concerns intentional care.

This proposed division requires at least one qualification. It is evident that intentional care will be a feature of identity-constituting care. Care is an ontological feature of persons, and this is manifested partly in the specific intentional cares they have – for example towards children or, if they are nurses, patients, or if they are social workers, clients, and so on.

With specific reference to the nursing context, we can set aside the notion of deep ontological care, and focus instead upon the second type of care, identity-constituting care, identified above. As noted, care in this sense is significant in that it points to an ontological role of care in the constitution of the person. This is a role such that nursing care of patients can usefully aim to discern such cares, what matters to the patient, in order to care for them.

Intentional care in nursing revisited

Given the relation between ontological and intentional care so far described, and given that intentional care requires appreciation of the plight of the patient, a term employed to describe such appreciation which can be coined here is 'sympathic awareness'. Note the *OED* definition of 'sympathy' as 'mental participation with another in his trouble...'. It is not being claimed here that this involves experiencing the patient's plight as he himself does, but rather that one has a conception of it in which one recognises the patient as vulnerable, as a being with the capacity to suffer, and with needs. On the basis of such sympathic awareness responses to suffering and unmet needs will be prompted.

We saw earlier that for Nortvedt such sympathic awareness necessarily has an emotional element. Roughly, such awareness itself involves a 'feeling' aspect; the patient's plight is 'felt for' at some level by the nurse. As in our earlier discussion, this seems a plausible view in relation to some kinds of nursing actions, for example responses to serious suffering, but is less plausible in relation to more mundane kinds of nursing actions.

However, as suggested earlier (Chapter 6), it is not implausible to suppose that our mode of being in the world has an inescapable, affective dimension to it. This strategy addresses the problem for Nortvedt's position caused by 'mundane' nursing acts, but as we saw earlier, it now follows that nursing acts have an emotional dimension because everything we do has such a dimension.

Before offering a conclusion, consider one more feature of caring acts. Consider again caring acts which are responses to serious suffering. From the moral perspective it may be claimed that sympathic awareness of such suffering generates a moral pull on the person who witnesses it. Even the examples of mundane nursing care can be said to exhibit a moral dimension. For even these are responses to vulnerability on the part of the nurse. So it is plausible to suppose they have a moral dimension.

Given this, we can advance the following tripartite analysis of acts of intentional caring. Acts of intentional caring necessarily involve:

(a) sympathic awareness of the plight of the patient;
(b) an emotional component – given acceptance of the existence of an emotional dimension to human being; and
(c) a response to what are perceived to be the needs of the patient.

Concerning (a), I have offered a brief description of this above, in the discussion of sympathic awareness. Concerning (b), to repeat, since all acts have an emotional element, so will all acts of intentional caring. Concerning (c), such a response is a plausible necessary condition of intentional caring acts. Also, given the moral dimension inherent in nursing actions, the idea of a moral pull can be recruited here: the plight of another exerts a moral pull on the nurse.

The relations between this account of intentional care and ontological care run as follows. With regard to the idea of care as having an emotional dimension, it was suggested that such a dimension is present in our mode of being in the world. So this ontological claim implies that all acts will have an affective dimension. So intentional care is necessarily permeated by this emotional dimension. As we have seen, appreciation of the identity-constituting sense of care is also crucial to intentional care. The affective dimension of our existence helps to explain this too. Given that we have an affective attitude to our self-project, one we feel committed to, this helps to explain further the impact of interpretations of symptoms by patients: any threat to the self-project perceived by the patient is likely to have an emotional aspect to it, as we have observed. Nursing care of such a patient seems plausibly to require appreciation of this.

With reference to the range of caring acts within the nursing context, for example from nursing responses to profound suffering, to nursing acts such as giving out routine medications, it has been claimed here that the threefold analysis of intentional caring acts can apply across this range.

It should be stressed, however, that each of the three components of intentional caring acts may be present in differing strengths. Thus, although sympathic awareness is a necessary condition of intentional caring, differences in nurses' sensitivity to this may entail differences in the degree to which differing nurses are able to appreciate the patient's plight. Similarly, although an emotional component will be present in intentional caring acts, this may be more strongly present in one nurse than another. People differ in their degree of emotional involvement and sensitivity, hence these kinds of differences are to be expected. A similar point can be made with reference to the idea of a moral pull. Although meeting the needs of others stems from such a pull, the pull may be felt more strongly by one nurse than by another. Thus although all three dimensions are present within intentional caring acts, they may be present in differing strengths in different individuals.

With regard to attempts to distinguish stronger and weaker forms of intentional caring (viz. de Raeve, 1996), the following claims can be advanced. Given that intentional caring within the nursing context requires a conception of the plight of the patient, it follows that strong and weak forms of such caring will similarly involve such a conception. An attempt to articulate the difference between strong and weak intentional caring as this might apply within the nursing context may exploit two ideas: that of a 'moral pull', and that of emotional involvement.

Concerning the idea of 'moral pull', the suggestion here would be that from the moral perspective, the patient's plight involves a moral pull at some level on the weak carer, but that this is not as weighty a pull as is exerted on the strong carer. Thus in a conflict between self-regarding and other-regarding acts, the weak carer is more likely to perform the self-regarding act than the strong carer.

With regard to emotional involvement, a similar story can be told. Given that weaker intentional caring has an emotional aspect, it can be anticipated that strong intentional caring brings with it a greater degree of emotional involvement with the person being cared for. It may be, of course, that this involvement is also a factor in the explanation of the difference in degrees of moral pull which the patient's plight exerts on the weak and strong carer. Thus the weightier moral pull felt by one person may be related to the greater level of emotional involvement.

It should be reiterated that intentional caring, even at the weaker end of the spectrum, will involve an emotional component; some level of feeling for the person being cared for will be present. Such feelings presuppose some division of phenomena into more and less salient features. To take an obvious example, in seeing a starving child what strikes one as salient is the suffering and misery endured by the child.

This is a mere sketch of how an attempt to fill out a distinction between strong and weak intentional caring might run. It is not my intention to provide such an account, only to indicate the kind of factors it might include.

The main point to take from this part of the discussion is that intentional caring within nursing, if it requires anything, must require a conception of the patient's plight; it was suggested further that such sensitivity provides the background against which caring practices such as nursing are intelligible.

This model of intentional caring relates to the ontological aspect of caring in the manner indicated earlier. That is to say, the patient's conception of his plight will be in terms of the significance of his symptoms for his own 'self-project'. Appreciation of this perspective on the symptoms is necessarily involved in intentional caring. Thus, intentional caring requires not simply appreciation of the plight of the patient considered in terms of suffering, but this appreciation has to be located within an understanding of the patient's conception of the significance of the symptoms for his own self-project. Of course, where patients do not have such a conception, for example due to coma, or severe cognitive problems, then appreciation at a more visceral, phenomenological level is all that is possible.

Summary

It has been proposed here that the type of ontological care most central to nursing is the identity-constituting kind described above. Recognition of the fact that persons are constituted by their cares and of the way in which symptoms of illness are interpreted in terms of these appears central to nursing. This parallels what was said concerning the narrative conception of the person in Chapter 5. Of course, to say this is not to say (absurdly) that the biological level of human existence need be of no concern to the nurse.

In relation to intentional care, it has been suggested that intentional care in the nursing context involves the following components: sympathic, emotional, moral (that is, as moral pull). And it has been suggested that such caring actions contribute to the ends of nursing by relieving suffering, making patients well and so on. Intentional care 'connects up' with identity-constituting care in that one is better equipped to relieve pain and suffering if one grasps the importance of identity-constituting care.

Thus, positions on ontological and intentional care have been described, as have their respective relations to nursing practice.

Three sets of considerations can now be signalled:

1. Modesty in relation to knowledge claims is generated by our discussion of propositional and practical knowledge.

2. Our discussion of persons indicates the centrality of interpretation to nursing. Patients interpret symptoms in terms of their significance for the pursuance of their self-projects. Nurses must try to glean some understanding of this. Patients seem in a privileged position when it comes to

determining the impact of illness on them. This applies at the phenomeno-logical level, and also in terms of the effect of illness on pursuance of a self-project. Any plausible account of nursing must respect these considerations.

3. Our account of care re-casts identity as pursuance of a self-project in terms of pursuance of what one cares about. This is simply a different way of expressing the same conception of persons described above (Chapter 5).

The discussion of care points to the centrality of the moral dimension to nursing. Acts of intentional care owe their intelligibility to a key ontological difference between humans and inanimate objects such that the former have the capacity to feel pain and to suffer, they are essentially vulnerable beings.

We turn in the next two chapters to look at the nature of nursing. Plainly any account of the nature of nursing must respect the conclusions arrived at so far. Any such account must, thus, be compatible with the accounts of knowledge, the person, and care developed here.

SUGGESTIONS FOR FURTHER READING

Care

Van Hooft's (1995) book is an accessible and fascinating discussion of care, in particular at the ontological level. Readers interested in a fuller discussion of this topic will find van Hooft of great interest. As mentioned in the text, the source of the onto-logical sense of care lies in the work of Heidegger (1962) so those with a serious interest should be guided to that. Heidegger's work is not easy. I find Mulhall (1996) a good, clear introduction to his work within *Being and Time*.

John Paley (2000) gives a very helpful account of Heidegger's sense of care and of attempts to employ this to develop an ethics of care. And Per Nortvedt's (1996) book provides a thorough, accessible discussion of an ethics of care in nursing.

8 *The nature of nursing (i): nursing as a science*

In this chapter and the next our focus lies on the nature of nursing. The present chapter assesses the claim that nursing is a science. Following clarification of that claim, we discuss the view of nursing as a science in terms of positivist, interpretivist, and realist philosophies of science. It is tentatively concluded that nursing is not a science. The justification for this conclusion stems largely from consideration of the kinds of phenomena which feature among the ends of nursing (pain, suffering, well-being and so on). It is not clear that these are such that they are 'fit' objects of scientific enquiry due to their experiential nature.

Clarifying the claim that nursing is a science

The claim that nursing is a science is encouraged by journal titles such as *Advances in Nursing Science*, and *Nursing Science Quarterly*, and it is specifically advanced in several places (see, Parse, 1987; Peplau, 1987; Orem, 1987). The claim is one supported with enthusiasm in some quarters (J. Clark, 1999), and dismay in others (L. Clarke, 1999).

The claim is also one in which I should declare a specific interest. The Centre for Philosophy and Health Care, within which I work is located within a 'School of Health Science'; it is involved, among other things, with the education of nurses. The clear implication of the title of the School seems to be that nursing figures within the health sciences, along with medicine, and that students who come to study nursing are engaged, primarily, in the study of a scientific discipline. That this is the case is explicitly declared in the title of a 'Doctorate in nursing science' to which I contribute some sessions on philosophy of nursing.

There seem two clear reasons why nursing might seek an alignment with science. The first relates to the prestigious nature of science. O'Hear writes 'There is no institution in the modern world more prestigious than science' (1989, p. 1). We should not, thus, be surprised that any discipline seeking such honorific status should seek to align itself with science.

The second reason stems from more than simply the desire for prestige. The reported prestige of science stems from its success in generating knowledge of the empirical world. Thus given acceptance of the view that it is preferable to base nursing practice upon that which is known as opposed to merely believed, then it seems rational to align nursing with science. So this reason for the alignment is based upon the view that one can nurse in a 'better way' if one has relevant knowledge, and one can obtain such knowledge by conducting nursing in a scientific manner.

Having identified these two grounds which can be appealed to to motivate an alignment with science, four preliminary points need to be made in order to clarify the focus of our inquiry.

Four preliminary points

1. The first preliminary point refers to a key constraint on our discussion. The claim that nursing is a science is a 'class inclusion' claim. It is a claim that nursing is a member of that class of activities which comprise the sciences (just as the statement 'A daffodil is a flower' is also a class inclusion claim). Those activities which are members of the class of sciences owe their membership of it by virtue of their possession of certain key characteristics (just as membership of the class of flowers is similarly so dependent upon the possession of certain key characteristics). Thus our strategy here will be as follows. We will attempt to identify characteristics reasonably supposed to be crucial for membership of the class of sciences. We then try to determine whether or not nursing is such that it is incompatible with the possession of such characteristics. So if we can identify a characteristic of science central to it and absent in nursing, we can show by this route that nursing and science differ. (This strategy exploits a logical rule relating to class membership such that membership of a class is dependent upon the possession of certain key characteristics.)

2. The second preliminary point raises a further constraint on our discussion. This is that no violence is done to the concepts of either nursing or science. In other words, that credible, recognisable pictures of each are what are claimed as related. Hence, the account of nursing that emerges after the identification with science has been made must be a credible, recognisable view of nursing. It must respect the three key elements of it as identified at the close of Chapter 7 relating to knowledge, persons and care. Second, of course, the same applies to science: the view of science with which nursing is said to be identical must be a credible conception of science. The account of science with which it is claimed nursing is identical must recognisably be science.

3. A third preliminary point runs thus. A major problem with the attempt to identify nursing with science is that it is possible to discern two main senses of the term 'science', one deriving from an ancient, Aristotelean conception of science, and the other a more restrictive modern view. The

Aristotelean view is one in which 'science' refers to any systematic body of knowledge (see *Ethics*, p. 174). Thus geometry, theology, botany, ethics and philosophy qualify as science.

Since this extreme view is so inclusive we can label it the 'broad view'. It seems reasonable to suppose that if someone claims nursing to be a science, and means science in this broad view, then their claim is not very interesting. Since it includes almost anything, it is not especially informative to be told that nursing is a science on this broad view of what is meant by the term 'science'.[1]

Opposed to this broad view is a narrower, more modern understanding of the term such that theology, ethics, and other bodies of knowledge would not be thought to count as science. I take it that when it is claimed that nursing is a science it is usually claimed to be so in this more restrictive, modern sense.

It should be stressed that it is the modern sense of 'science' which has the positive connotations that have led nurses to claim nursing to be a science. For it is science in the modern sense of the term which is associated with successful knowledge gathering and which nursing (among other disciplines, for example medicine) seeks to emulate or adopt.

4. The fourth and final preliminary point is this. The fact that a discipline employs the findings of science is not sufficient for it to be the case that that discipline is itself a science. A sculptor may use the findings of materials science in order to determine which material to use for her sculpture, but it need not follow from this that sculpting is a science. So although nurses undoubtedly use the findings of science – for example chemistry, physics, biology – in their work it need not follow from this that nursing is itself a science.

These four preliminary points all seem central to bear in mind when assessing the case for the claim that nursing is a science.

Prior to considering three scientific movements within nursing, I would like first to try to signal some obstacles that will need to be overcome if the claim that nursing is a science is to be sustained.

Two prima-facie obstacles

First, it seems that science is essentially a descriptive enterprise. The business of the natural sciences is to describe the natural world, of astronomy to describe the heavens, of psychology to describe the processes of human cognition and emotion and so on, of sociology to describe social relations and institutions.[2]

In contrast to the essentially descriptive nature of science, nursing is essentially normative (see, for example, Bishop and Scudder, 1997). This normativity can be illustrated in two senses. First, nurses aim to bring about certain kinds of states rather than others, for example the relief of suffering. This is in contrast to science where what are aimed at are true descriptions of the world. There is no aim to bring about one class of true descriptions as opposed to another class. As long as a description is accurate, the scientist has done her job. In contrast, the nurse has to bring about states of a specific kind.

Relatedly, whereas the ends of the scientist are primarily descriptive any plausible candidates for the ends of nursing will be evaluative in nature. These will include concepts such as relieving suffering or pain, promoting well-being, quality of life and autonomy and so on. These are inherently evaluative concepts: they are defined by reference to human values. This is not the case with the descriptive concepts which figure in the ends of science. As argued, its ends are to describe the world. Thus a statement such as 'There are nine planets in the solar system' counts as an example of a statement which meets the ends of science. It contains no evaluative elements.

A second prima-facie obstacle to the identification of nursing and science is this one. Description of the world within science is itself of *intrinsic* significance. As put previously, the scientist has done her job when she has given us a true description of some part of the world. Contrast this with any description of a patient's condition, for example 'Smith's temperature is normal/abnormal'. The whole point of seeking Smith's temperature is inseparable from evaluative concerns. If Smith's temperature is abnormal, is this affecting his well-being? Is he suffering? Can we put a stop to this? If Smith's temperature is normal, we need not be concerned about it, he is not in danger, at least from any health threatening conditions which are generated by abnormal temperature. The descriptions of Smith are significant only given the evaluative ends aimed at in nursing. Within the nursing domain, descriptions of patient's conditions, or of the mechanisms by which drugs are effective, are of essentially *instrumental* significance only. Such descriptions are means towards fulfilment of the ends of nursing Smith. This is not so in science. Descriptions there are of intrinsic, not necessarily instrumental significance.

These two prima-facie obstacles are attempts to show that the class inclusion claim 'nursing is a science' is bound to fail. For we seem to have identified two key characteristics of membership of the class of sciences which nursing, due to its nature, lacks. It seems to follow nursing cannot be a science.

A response

In response to these obstacles it is then often claimed that nursing is an *applied* science. Or, indeed, a science of the application of applied science (for example in the sense that, say, using a sophisticated wound dressing is applying applied science – the applied science being the process leading to the development of the dressing). Of course this has to amount to more than the claim that nurses use the findings of science. As noted above, that a discipline employs the findings of science is not sufficient to show the discipline to be a science.

Suppose this 'something more' can be shown. If so, the second obstacle seems to be overcome. For in an applied science, scientific findings are employed for instrumental purposes. For example, a description of the properties of steel can be recruited, instrumentally, towards the end of building a bridge.

If in saying nursing is an applied science it is meant that the findings of science are instigated *in a scientific manner*, so to speak, that is, in a specifiable manner, then perhaps nursing is an applied science such as civil engineering.

But a crucial difference remains. Nursing actions are answerable to subjective considerations in a way in which applied sciences are not. The fact of whether or not a bridge is a good bridge can be determined by objective criteria. Does the bridge reach the other side of the river? Does it bear the weight necessary for it to be used? Can it withstand wind and rain and so on?

The question of whether or not a pattern of nursing interventions is a good one cannot be determined wholly by objective criteria. As we saw in our discussions of narrative identity (Chapter 5) and identity-constituting care (Chapter 7) the nurse has to be sensitive to the patient's own perspective on his predicament. Thus the views of the patient on the matter seem central to the question of whether or not nursing interventions have been 'good'. And what 'good' amounts to here seems bound to the patient's perspective on the interventions. This is in terms of how the patient actually *feels* (that is, is the pain relieved and so on), and also of the patient's view of the impact of his condition upon his self-project. Bishop and Scudder (1991, p. 31) for example, emphasise the importance of 'unique personal relations' in nursing. There is no echo of this in bridge building, or engineering and so on. There is no requirement to consider that materially equivalent items (for example individual pieces of copper) should be handled differently. There is such a consideration in nursing, and it is central to nursing, as our narrative account of the person shows.

Also, what if it were accepted that those who apply the findings of applied science are themselves scientists by virtue of this fact. This would appear to show that the labourers who construct a bridge (for example bricklayers) are themselves scientists – in that they apply applied science. Such a view seems deeply implausible.

Lastly, there is a further more obvious difference between nursing and applied sciences such as engineering. The objects of the applied sciences lack subjectivity. The objects of nursing do not.

It may be objected that this response ignores the human sciences in which phenomena such as 'meaning' and privately experienced feelings are considered fit objects of scientific investigation. But even in these human sciences such enquiry differs crucially from nursing. For as seen, knowledge is obtained in nursing for instrumental reasons. This is a necessary truth about nursing, but is not when considered in relation to knowledge gathering in the human sciences. There knowledge is valued for its own sake. Further, as our discussion of care shows, if anything is true of nursing it is that it has a moral dimension, and does so *necessarily*. Such a dimension is at most a contingent feature of science, natural or human, applied or pure.

To summarise: at first it seemed that nursing could not be a science since knowledge obtained in science seems essentially descriptive. Knowledge obtained in nursing, by contrast, is primarily for instrumental purposes. But as we saw, this will not serve to distinguish nursing from applied sciences. In these knowledge is used instrumentally.

But before we accept that nursing is an applied science some qualifications and further grounds for doubt need to be rehearsed. First, nursing involves the application of applied science, as in, say, the application of a sophisticated wound dressing. The dressing is the product of applied science, which the nurse makes use of. Second, that a person is applying applied science need not entail they are themselves engaged in science – recall the 'bricklayer' example.

In the light of these qualifications how should we now regard the claim that nursing is a science, an applied science? There seem to be three grounds for scepticism about such a claim. First, in nursing it is necessary to treat individual patients differently, even if they are 'physically equivalent' in, say, having the same problem in biological terms. But in applied science it seems crucial to treat all samples of kind in the same way. The pharmacist developing a new drug assumes each sample of the relevant chemical ingredient has the same properties and hence that all samples of the drug will behave in the same way. The same applies in relation to, say, the development of prostheses. The person developing these assumes each sample of the relevant material will possess the same properties (for example pliability, strength and so on). This is broadly the point made above by Bishop and Scudder.

Second, related to the last objection, the objects of applied science lack subjectivity and must do so. It 'works on' inanimate objects.

Third, as we saw, there are objective criteria available in order to determine whether or not the ends of applied science have been met (for example to determine whether or not a bridge is a good bridge). This is not the case in nursing. The question of how a patient feels is accessible to them in a way which makes it the case that it is problematic to determine objectively whether or not the ends of nursing have been achieved.

So, with these preliminary skirmishes completed, let us now consider further the claim that nursing is a science. It should be said that our skirmishes militate against the likelihood of this, but it will prove instructive to try to pursue the question.

We will look at three strategies for 'knowledge gathering' within nursing, each of which has been claimed to capture what is distinctive of science. The three strategies are positivism, interpretivism and realism.

We saw that the claim that nursing is a science must be subject to two constraints, one relating to 'class inclusion' claims; and the other that in pursuing the claim no violence is done to the concepts of either nursing or science. In other words, that credible, recognisable pictures of each are what are claimed as related.

As will be seen, of the three approaches we consider positivism seems to fail to live up to either constraint: it provides neither a satisfactory account of science nor of nursing. Interpretivism best matches nursing, but it is not clear that it matches science. Realism, as will also be seen, matches science, but does it match nursing? I will argue that it does not in at least one key respect. It should be said at the outset of our discussion of these three movements within philosophy of science that it is deeply problematic to characterise nursing in terms of any of them. For they are primarily strategies for knowledge gathering. As such they cannot hope to provide an exhaustive account of nursing for, as we saw, nursing involves more than gathering knowledge it involves acting on it in ways which further the ends of nursing.

Positivism

In the last section we noted three views on how best to acquire scientific knowledge of the world. The first of these is positivism. The term originates in the work of Comte (1830) and signifies the attempt to place scientific findings on a firm or 'positive' basis. Standardly, such a positive basis is taken to be sense experience, empirical evidence. On the basis of such evidence, anchored in sense experience, theories can be constructed in order to explain the happenings in the world. (Strictly speaking positivism is a collection of positions (see Halfpenny, 1982) but for our purposes certain key commitments can be singled out.)

Reasonably enough, since it is thought that this is the most favourable means of obtaining knowledge, it is proposed that the positivist method be adopted by all sciences, so-called methodological monism. Thus, on this view, a discipline is a science if and only if it subscribes to the tenets of positivism. Foremost among these tenets is the view that claims be grounded in that which is positively the case, that which rests upon sensory evidence.[3]

Thus if the positivist conception of science is correct, the claim that nursing is a science can be evaluated by examination of the approaches to knowledge gathering which are current within nursing.

However, as is now extremely widely recognised the tenets of positivism are themselves dubious, especially as they apply to the study of human beings (see, for example, Bhaskar, 1975, 1989). A key problem centres on the appeal to sensory evidence as a 'positive' basis for theories. This presupposes that descriptions of sensory experiences, such as reports of what one observes (observation statements) are theory free. And, hence, that a sharp distinction is possible between observational statements and theoretical statements. But this claim is now thought to be mistaken. The counter view is that observation statements themselves are 'tainted' with theory. To see this, consider a statement such as 'That's a glass of water'.

This presupposes ontological claims such that water exists, that glass exists, that glass is transparent. And perhaps less obviously, it presupposes that the glass has not spontaneously come into existence that very second, but has endured over some lengthier time span. Still more abstractly, the statement presupposes that things exist in time and space – that is, that the glass of water has a spatio-temporal location. Thus, if these presuppositions are reasonably characterised as theoretical, the observation statement just given is heavily imbued with theory. Of course it may be denied that these presuppositions are in fact theoretical in nature. Yet, it seems plausible to suppose they are: they are part of the theory we learn in learning the English language, and in learning how to refer to things around us. In other words, in learning our language we learn one particular way of organising the world around us. This is also, of course, informed by our senses which present the world to us in one way rather than another. For example, if we could 'see' heat, a further dimension of the world would apparently be evident in our observation reports. (This too, of course, would introduce a further theoretical element to such reports, for example regarding the existence and nature of heat.)

Also, it is widely accepted that what is 'seen' by observers is not independent of cultural factors. For example, in cultures where there is no tradition of representing three-dimensional objects by two-dimensional drawings, such phenomena are not seen as they are by subjects from cultures where representation of three-dimensional objects on a two-dimensional plane is prevalent. (See Chalmers, 1982, p. 25.)

So the idea that there is this unpolluted basis for theoretical claims can be shown to be highly dubious, and unsurprisingly, attempts to align nursing with a positivist account of science have met with strong resistance. This has come not only from those sympathetic to the idea of nursing as a science (for example Gortner, 1990; Schumacher and Gortner, 1992) but also from those who appear more cautious about such an alignment (for example Benner, 1985).

This objection to positivism strikes at its very core. It shows positivism not to be compatible with an adequate account of science, and so fails to meet the second condition of adequacy noted at the start of this discussion.

It may be supposed there is no point in discussing the position further. However, it is my view that there is something instructive in pursuing, in particular, the question of the inapplicability of positivism to the nursing context. The reason is that some of the problems which arise in applying it, arise when attempts are made to apply other approaches. Thus we now turn to discuss briefly why the possibility of an adequate positivist account of nursing is remote.

As we heard, sensory evidence is the claimed bedrock for scientific data according to the positivist. This boils down to the view that there is no legitimate place in science for data which are essentially private. That is to say, two 'perspectives' from which data are presented can be discerned. The first-person perspective is the perspective we all have on our own mental experiences. This perspective, it seems, is unique to each one of us.

The third-person perspective presents data which are public, or accessible to all observers. For example, a chair in the middle of the room is accessible to all of us from the third-person perspective. Contrast this with one's own current feelings and thoughts, these seem accessible to us in a radically different way, they seem essentially 'private', not public.

The positivist emphasis upon empirical data may be appropriate if the relevant data are publicly accessible – for example the movements of tides, planets, a patient's temperature, weight and so on. But what if the data we are interested in are data primarily accessible from the first-person perspective?

This range of data presents a further serious problem for the applicability of positivist method: it seems essentially private, not publicly accessible, hence difficulties concerning verification and falsification of hypotheses arise. And worse, we standardly take it to be the case that the first-person perspective is one which is particularly authoritative: surely we as individuals are best placed to know what we are currently feeling and thinking, and we might not choose to divulge this to anyone else.

This particular problem in applying positivist method to nursing seems especially significant. For much nursing research seeks to focus on such apparently private data: the 'felt' or phenomenological experiences of patients and nurses and so on. And there is a good reason for this focus. The states which characterise the ends of nursing seem primarily to have a crucial phenomenological element to them – well-being, pain, suffering, quality of life and so on. These are key aspects of the plight of the patient, the morally salient features of the patient's predicament which prompt the moral response of the nurse.

Finally, we noted in our discussion of persons that their acts stem from their own conception of their predicament, and their goals. Such conceptions are not necessarily evident in the way in which positivism seems to require. There is a gap between thought and behaviour such that one cannot identify the two. For example, behaving as though one is in pain differs from actually being in pain. Indeed Halfpenny observes that positivism seems to require behaviourism (1982, p. 91).

As our discussion of persons and care suggest (Chapters 6 and 7), the attempt to interpret the patient's conception of their situation is crucial to nursing. This, once more, does not seem simply manifest in the patient's behaviour, but requires interpretive skill on the part of the nurse.

So the private, subjective nature of much of the phenomena of concern to nurses presents a clear problem for the applicability of positivism to nursing. The need to interpret what patients say and do also presents problems. This seems to require the nurse to 'go beyond' what a patient may actually say, and speculate upon what the patient really means, or whether they indeed mean what they say. And lastly, nursing has an inherent moral dimension to it. Yet moral properties do not seem 'open to view' in the way positivism requires. For example, can one 'see' that an act of truthtelling is good or bad? So this dimension, crucial to nursing, also seems difficult to accommodate within a positivist perspective.

Thus it is reasonable to conclude that positivism fails to meet both our conditions of adequacy. It fails to match a credible view of science, and fails also to match a credible account of nursing. There could not be a positivist account of nursing which was recognisable as nursing.

Interpretivism

The subjective, 'first-person' nature of phenomena of key concern to nursing, the all-pervasiveness of interpretation, and recognition of the moral dimension of nursing led to what we can term an 'interpretive turn' within nursing. Benner and Wrubel go so far as to describe their approach to nursing as an 'interpretive theory of nursing' (1989, p. 7).

Interpretivism refers to a movement within philosophy of science which, as may be anticipated, points to the necessity of interpreting phenomena, notably when engaged in the investigation of human action and other social practices. Thus, in contrast with the positivist picture rehearsed above, it is presumed that the study of humans will require different methods than those appropriate for the study of the natural world.

Indeed, a distinction is commonly made between the natural and the human sciences (see, for example, Hempel, 1966; Hiley et al., 1991). The grounds for this are similar to those rehearsed in our discussion of positivism. The presence of subjectivity, meaning and values in the study of humans seems to entail that study of them will differ importantly from study of inanimate things – rocks, planets, tides and so on. As Bhaskar puts it, the natural sciences are characterised by subject–object relations, and the human sciences by subject–subject relations (1989, p. 21).

Interpretivists suppose that interpretation is required in the study of humans. So, it is implied, the recognition of the layers of complexity involved in studying humans need not itself preclude scientific scrutiny of human life. Given this, what I propose to do now is to say more about this 'interpretive turn' and then return to the question of the taking of the turn and scientific status.

As noted, this 'turn' has culminated in the proposal of an 'interpretive theory of nursing' (Benner and Wrubel, 1989, p. 7). The approach encourages a centring of attention on subjective phenomena such as the experiences of pain, stress, and the interpretations of both patients and nurses of the situations within which they are embedded.

In justification of this, as we have seen, the prevalence of interpretation within the nursing context is easy to point to. Judgements that a patient is anxious, aggressive, or in need of reassurance, all presuppose interpretation by the nurse. Similarly, a decision by a nurse to alert a doctor to a patient's sudden rise in blood pressure equally involves an interpretation on the part of the nurse. In fact, it seems trivially true that all actions derive from interpretations, and hence that all actions within the nursing context do so too.

As we saw in Chapters 5 and 7 above, less trivially, patients' interpretations of their predicaments can be of deep significance. This is especially important when they become ill.

It should be stressed that when Benner and Wrubel describe nurses as interpreting the utterances and actions of patients it need not be supposed that they go through a series of conscious steps of reasoning. On the contrary, typically, such interpretations arise without such a process – this applies especially to the expert nurse (see Benner, 1984; and Chapter 4 above). With these points in mind we now move on to offer two brief comments on this turn, and then to look at some criticisms of it.

Comments on the interpretive turn

It is a considerable merit of the interpretive turn that it stresses the importance of aspects of health care which the standard, positivist account either excludes, or disregards. As noted, such aspects include the subjective experience of illness, the patient's conception of his predicament, and the moral dimension of health care work. So a merit of the interpretive turn in the context of health care is the proper incorporation of subjectivity, meaning, and value.

More critically, it may be said that some violence is done to the concept of interpretation by proponents of the interpretive turn. Pre-philosophically, we suppose that an interpretation on our part requires a conscious act of interpretation. But due, largely, to Heidegger and Kuhn, 'interpretation' has come to be used in such a way that if a view could be otherwise, then that view comprises an interpretation (see Heidegger, 1962, p. 190; Kuhn, 1970; Mulhall, 1996, p. 86). (Hence, similarly, any observation statement counts as an interpretation on this line of thought.)

So on this account of interpretation, in effect, any judgement is an interpretation. Any world view, scientific theory or specific commonsense judgement involves an interpretation (this is 'hermeneutic universalism' Shusterman, 1991, p. 102). However, in spite of the merits of the turn, and the question of its distortion of ordinary linguistic usage, there are some serious difficulties with the turn to intepretivism which need signalling.

Some problems with the interpretive turn

What if a dispute arises as to how to interpret a set of behaviours (or indeed the body of a PVS patient (Gadow, 1989)). Suppose one nurse interprets a patient's actions as a sign of distress, inviting further involvement with the nurse, and another interprets these same actions as signs of rejection of nursing involvement – as expressing a wish to be left alone. Respecting the wishes of this patient requires interpretation of what they are. Suppose he says 'Go away, leave me alone', it seems to me that this still could be interpreted in either of the ways just described (for example 'deep down he just wants to talk').

To give another example. Prior to her death Diana, Princess of Wales, gave a TV interview describing some of the details of her life as the wife of Prince Charles. Many interpreted the interview as a cry for help, or as an outpouring of sorrow. Many others interpreted the interview as a cynical piece of media manipulation. Who is right?

Further, along these same lines, it is a well-known point of Wittgenstein's that interpretations can also be interpreted, and so on and so on (1953, for example, para. 217). When does one stop the process of interpreting?

Second, and related to the last area of concern, it is a tenet of psychoanalysis that on a significant number of occasions we do not know what we are really thinking. For example, we may not know what our 'real' motivations are for becoming a healthcare professional, or for disliking a particular patient, or colleague. Yet, Benner and Wrubel's account of nursing supposes that the nurse must grasp 'the meaning of the illness for the person [that is, the patient]' (1989, p. 9). This supposes that such a meaning is evident to the patient, and there are Freudian grounds for being suspicious of that supposition. So this last objection queries that people do actually know what they think.

Relatedly, at the societal level, there are grounds to doubt that people's own interpretations of their actions are accurate. For example, those working within the field of Soviet psychiatry may have supposed that their work was to rehabilitate mentally ill people. Yet others may plausibly interpret their work as primarily involving the suppression of dissidence (hence diagnoses of 'ideological intoxication'). So at the level of the individual and at the level of social groups there are grounds to doubt the supposition that interpretations are always accurate, such interpretations may be distorted by ideological inculcation or 'false consciousness' (for example Bhaskar, 1989, p. 21).

A third objection is similar to the last in that it queries the supposition that people know what they think, but it queries it in a different way. It is standardly claimed within philosophy of language that a person's use of language is answerable to public usage (Wittgenstein, 1953; Burge, 1979). This is evidenced by the possibility of misuse of language. The possibility of such misuse, it is claimed, presupposes public standards for correct usage. It seems to follow from this that descriptions of one's own mental states are not, then, necessarily correct. For example, if a person mistakenly thinks arthritis occurs in muscles, in his statement 'I have arthritis in my thigh' the meaning of the term 'arthritis' is fixed by the relevant linguistic community. So it is not even clear that the person can be said to know what they are thinking.

Hence although the interpretive approach to nursing may represent a more adequate one than the positivist approach, it too seems beset with some deep and difficult problems. Those just described seem serious. Other concerns, omitted here, but which also seem serious include the complaint that the interpretive turn in nursing has led to a neglect of the bodily element of care, or at least, to a relegation of its significance (for example, Dunlop, 1986; Paley, 1999). The charge is that nurses have focused so much on interpretation construed as psychological interpretation, that the equally important domain of bodily care and interpretation of bodily factors is being overlooked.

Interpretivism is also charged with embracing relativism and subjectivism (S. Wainwright, 1997). The complaint is that within the approach, all inter-pretations are considered equally legitimate; there are no grounds to regard one interpretation as superior in any way to another rival interpretation. This criticism takes us to the question of whether, in taking the interpretivist turn, nursing can retain any claim to be a science.

In relation to our two conditions of adequacy, consider again whether interpretivism sits with an adequate account of nursing. With reservations just noted it can.

But is it compatible with an adequate account of *science*? The criticism that it is not has been voiced in recent years (see, for example, Schumacher and Gortner, 1992; S. Wainwright, 1997; Hussey, 2000). The criticism concerns the kinds of situations in which there are rival interpretations of a phenomenon (recall the 'Go away, leave me alone' example). In order to meet the require-ment of matching a credible conception of science, interpretivists must allow that some interpretations are 'better than' others. From the realist perspective, true interpretations are 'best' since they match reality, match what is the case. Thus realist critics of interpretivism point out that to match a credible account of science, interpretivism must embrace realism. For, the view that there are better or worse interpretations, the criticism runs, presupposes there is a fact of the matter, that is, that there is something to be correct or incorrect *about*. Thus a *credible* form of interpretivism must embrace realism, or so it is argued.

However, at least some interpretivists appear to wish to avoid any commit-ment to realism. For example, Benner's own view seems explicitly to reject realism. She seems explicit that realism is false, 'The underlying assumption [in interpretive phenomenology] is that no one precise story exists, but rather multiple stories…' (1994, p. 111). So it appears true of Benner's form of interpretivism at least that she wishes to avoid realism.

Of course it remains open to interpretivists to try to maintain that realism can be avoided. But even if this move were to succeed, this would then call into question the credibility of regarding interpretivism as a science. For, it is claimed, science is inherently realist.

(Realism is understood here as the view that there is in fact a way the world is – an ontological claim. Science seeks to describe that way. Similarly, in the social realm too, there are facts of the matter. Thus in a dispute between two interpreters, there is something about which they are disputing, and which, were it known, could settle their dispute.)

Thus in so far as interpretivism refrains from realism, claims for an interpretivist science seem in jeopardy. However, it should be said that there is no *necessary* incompatibility between interpretivism and realism. Surely, it remains open to the interpretivist simply to accept the realist's ontological claim. It is possible to do this, and at the same time to accept the complexity of the phenomena with which nursing is primarily concerned – meaning, subjectivity and value.

So an attempt to align an interpretivist account of nursing with science could be salvaged without too much difficulty.

Moreover, it seems clear that there is a role for the provision of evidence within interpretivism, and thus that in a conflict between interpretations, evidence can be offered in favour of one and against another. It is unlikely that such evidence will be absolutely decisive, recall our discussions on knowledge. But nonetheless it seems that evidence such as a patient's past acts in similar situations could reasonably be appealed to in support of one interpretation over another competing one.

In an attempt to offer some guidance on the thorny question of how to choose between rival interpretations, Benner herself suggests that 'imaginative dwelling' (1994, p. 99) in the perspective of the other person is required. Of course, this is not unproblematic; understanding people from a culture radically different from one's own limits the possibility of imaginative dwelling. And what if researcher A, as a result of imaginative dwelling supports interpretation *x*, while researcher B, as a result of imaginative dwelling, concludes in favour of interpretation *y*? This is a serious difficulty for this approach, but the fact that a role can be envisaged for evidence suggests that no fatal consequences for an alignment with science need follow from our taking the interpretive turn. (Recall again here the 'virtues' proposed by Quine and Ullian. These too might usefully be invoked in order to try to evaluate competing interpretations.)

So the alignment with interpretivism in so far as it retains a key role for evidence and for realism (assuming these to be indispensable characteristics of science) generates no fatal problems for the attempt to be a science either. A role for empirical evidence need not be jettisoned; nor need a commitment to ontological realism.

At least one further source of difficulty can be envisaged however, concerning the idea of generalisability. This seems a key requirement of scientific claims. Thus in relation to the natural world, what is true of one sample of chlorine can be generalised to other samples. And to a less impressive degree this is also true in the human sciences. But in so far as Benner's interpretivism focuses on the individual nature of responses to symptoms of illness, then the possibility of generalising any findings seems called into question. From the fact that one patient responded well to one pattern of interventions by a nurse, it does not follow that other patients will, even if they have similar physical problems. For as we have seen, what is crucial is how patients themselves interpret their symptoms. And it seems very problematic to make generalisations within the interpretive approach (that is, to suppose that because patient A interpreted her symptoms in way *w*, then patient B will also; this is the case even if A and B have identical physical problems).

And yet, of course, the claim that patients will interpret symptoms in terms of their narratives is also a generalisation. So there is generalisation within interpretivism as Benner exploits this. (This tension between general and particular is one we take up in the final chapter.)

So two aspects of interpretivism which seem reasonable features of scientific enquiry are not jettisoned within interpretivism: the appeal to evidence and generalisability *at some level*. And, as noted, commitment to realism is not incompatible with interpretivism. So the interpretivist has room to manoeuvre here.

Thus, interpretivism can meet our two conditions of adequacy. It can sit with a credible picture of science (with suitable adjustments), and can sit with an apparently credible picture of nursing (that is, in which interpretation plays a central role).

Nonetheless, concerns with the adequacy of the interpretivist turn have led some commentators to argue for the adoption of a form of realism, of the kind propounded by Roy Bhaskar (1975, 1989), Schumacher and Gortner (1992), S. Wainwright (1997), Hussey (2000).

Realism

It should be repeated at the outset of our discussion here that there is no *necessary* incompatibility between interpretivism and (ontological) realism. The interpretivist can allow that there really is a fact of the matter, in interpretations, even if this could never be known. One of the important points brought out by realists within philosophy of science is that the intelligibility of enquiry seems to presuppose realism, that is, to presuppose that there really is a fact of the matter.

It is important to stress, however, that one can accept this ontological claim, and at the same time be sceptical that we could ever have knowledge of what is 'the fact of the matter'.

It may be that, as with our discussion of knowledge, the best we can do is opt for the interpretation which seems to us most plausible given what we currently take to be true, and given our sensitivity to the fact that our view of interpretations will never be neutral. All descriptions come from within some theory or other. So, there is always the possibility that a new hypothesis (that is, interpretation) will be resisted on the grounds that it conflicts with an interpretation which is currently held strongly and which is taken to be extremely plausible. For example, the hypothesis that stomach ulcers have a bacterial cause was resisted for years on the grounds that it conflicted with the then widely accepted view that the stomach is a sterile area. It was thought that due to its acidity, bacteria could not survive long enough in it to cause ulcers (see Thagard, 1998), but this view was later overturned.

Bhaskar's approach is to take as his starting point that science takes place, and to try to deduce what must be the case for this starting point to obtain. This is his so-called transcendental strategy: given that a social practice *x* occurs, one seeks to deduce 'necessary conditions for the particular activity' (1989, p. 7). Also: 'one assumes at the outset the intelligibility of science (or rather of a few generally recognised scientific activities) and asks explicitly what the world must be like for those activities to be possible' (ibid., p. 8).

The adoption of this strategy leads Bhaskar to conclude that the intelligibility of natural science presupposes a world capable of existing independently of the existence of humans. It is this world which scientists investigate, try to gather knowledge of. And, moreover, it is a world with 'ontological depth' (ibid., p. 12). In other words, surface phenomena we experience are generated by structures and mechanisms which are not immediately presented to us. Scientists work to uncover these.

Of course the social realm is not independent of the existence of humans in the way in which the natural realm is. But nonetheless, the same claim concerning ontological depth can be sustained. In other words, in the social realm there are structures which need to be invoked in the explanation of social phenomena. These include, of course, social structures (for example institutions of government, the health service, the education system and so on). Thus, an explanation of why it is that people work may make reference to the particular economic structures and institutions in the society in question. And, as with the natural world, it is held that appearance and reality differ. Hence, a subject may be mistaken about the real reasons for their actions.

The defining feature of Bhaskar's approach is described by him as follows: 'On this transcendental realist view of science, then, its essence lies in the *movement* at any one level from knowledge of manifest phenomena to knowledge of the structures that generate them' (1989, p. 13). Scientific enquiry, by definition, involves an attempt to show how appearances ('manifest phenomena' (ibid.)) are generated by underlying structures. In other words, how appearance relates to reality. It seems reasonable to conclude from Bhaskar's view that any possible object of scientific enquiry must be such that it can be analysed in terms of such an appearance/reality distinction.

Thus in his view the world has 'ontological depth' (1989, p. 12); the way the world appears may differ from how it is really. And, phenomena at the 'manifest' level are generated by structures at a deeper ontological level. Hence, for example, the solidity of a table is 'generated' by its composition at the micro-level; and a person's fainting (a manifest phenomenon) is generated by underlying structures, for example, which lead to low blood pressure, and bring about the person's faint.

With specific reference to the human sciences, Bhaskar writes:

> the predicates that appear in the explanation of social phenomena will be different from those that appear in natural scientific explanations, and the procedures used to establish them will in certain vital respects be different too (being contingent upon, and determined by, the properties of the objects under study); but the principles that govern their production will remain substantially the same (1989, p. 20).

With regard to the 'predicates', explanations within the human sciences will invoke different terms (predicates), for example those of agency, person, belief, desire, to the predicates which will figure in natural scientific explanations.

And, with regard to the 'procedures' involved in scientific enquiry, Bhaskar allows that these will differ due to the difference in the extent to which interpretation pervades the two areas of enquiry. It is allowed that interpretation is present in both the natural and the human sciences, but that a further layer of interpretive complexity pervades the latter.

Hence, it may be worth stressing that Bhaskar's pursuit of methodological monism is not driven by a reductionist view of humans (1989, pp. 2, 81), nor a reductionist view of societies (ibid., p. 25).

Lastly, with regard to the 'principles' of scientific explanation, for Bhaskar these will be shared by both modes of enquiry. For example, the summary statement of Bhaskar's conception of science quoted earlier can be seen to apply to the human sciences. That is, a difference between manifest and underlying phenomena is retained, and so too is the view that manifest phenomena are 'generated' by underlying phenomena – for example intentions, or some other explanatory category (for example 'social forms' (1989, p. 25) or structures).

It is worth stressing further, that Bhaskar's approach is realist in the sense that the generative structures which it is the business of the scientist to uncover are, in fact real (for example 1989, p. 14). The existence of such entities/structures is posited in the most robust sense possible: their existence is not dependent upon merely instrumental grounds, for example.

In summary, and oversimplifying a little, the position Bhaskar sets out is distinct from both positivism and interpretivism, and is in fact critical of each of these approaches. Among other more sophisticated objections against positivism, Bhaskar rejects the positivist view of a separation between theoretical and observation statements. And also he rejects the positivist view that the 'real world' is simply that which can be experienced. For him, as noted earlier, the world has an ontological depth which is ignored in positivism (1989, p. 15).

Against interpretivism, oversimplifying for present purposes, Bhaskar rejects the view that subjects' own interpretations are always correct (1989, p. 21). (A criticism to which Benner's line seems vulnerable (1985, p. 6).) As noted above, it is feasible that subjects may be mistaken about their real motivations for acting in one way rather than another. They may have been hoodwinked by ideological forces, or be under hypnosis, or there may be other reasons (see our earlier criticisms of interpretivism). And of course, insofar as interpretivism involves rejection of realism, it is vulnerable to serious objection from Bhaskar's viewpoint. (See Chapter 4 of Bhaskar, 1989 for the full details of his case against interpretivism.)

It is not necessary for my purposes to provide further details of Bhaskar's realism. What I intend to do is to assume its coherence and robustness as a philosophy of science. Then, against proponents of its applicability to nursing, I will describe a serious reservation concerning its applicability to this domain.

Against the realist turn in nursing

A first problem stems from the essentially normative nature of nursing. The applicability of realism to the natural and social realms seems relatively unproblematic. A condition of adequacy on realist accounts of phenomena within these realms is that they properly describe such phenomena, that is, that the relations between manifest phenomena and underlying structures are correctly characterised.

But this essentially descriptive task does not straightforwardly map on to the nursing context. As noted, realist theories of the natural and social realms are essentially descriptive. But any theory of nursing must involve a specification of its ends and means, and as will now be shown, that is where difficulties for the realist programme emerge.

Although the precise nature of the ends of nursing may be disputed, there is broad agreement concerning the range of possible solutions to the question. Ends such as promoting well-being, or quality of life, relieving pain and suffering will figure in any acceptable account of the ends of nursing. These ends plainly have a subjective component within them. This is evident in that the question of whether a patient's well-being, or quality of life has improved or deteriorated is necessarily answerable to that patient's own view of the matter. The same point can be made, perhaps more forcefully, by reference to the end of relieving pain and suffering. The question of whether or not a person's suffering has been relieved is necessarily answerable to that person's own view of the matter; perhaps, more strongly, it can even be claimed that the answer to such a question is uniquely determined by that person's judgement.

The difference here between the nursing context and the explanation of social action seems explicable in terms of the relative importance of phenomenological data. In the explanation of social action, it is perfectly conceivable that, for reasons of 'false consciousness' (an extreme example being a subject who acts under hypnosis) a subject may be unaware of the genuine explanation of his actions. Hence there is an epistemic gap between what a subject believes to be his reason for acting, and what is really the case. This is the gap which Bhaskar exploits to show that human science really is science (see section on 'Realism' above and the quote from Bhaskar, 1989, p. 13). But there does *not* seem a comparable gap in relation to phenomenological data: there does not seem a comparable gap between thinking that one is in pain, and really being in pain; or between thinking that one is suffering less, and really suffering less. Hence it seems to me that the particular nature of nursing (and health care work generally) poses a serious problem for the adequacy of the realist turn in nursing.

In other words, Bhaskar's realist conception of science requires an epistemic gap between how things seem – manifest phenomena – and the underlying phenomena which 'generate' manifest phenomena. But in the case of phenomena such as being in pain or suffering, no such epistemic gap is present. Therefore, a serious difficulty for the applicability of the realist programme to nursing seems to have been identified.

Obviously, the realist scientist can tell us whether or not a person has a particular virus or lesion within his bodily system. And it may be that there is a fact of the matter in relation to questions such as 'Is this patient's suffering worse than it was earlier?' But the objection raised here is that insofar as realism requires a distinction between how things appear and how things really are, it does not seem applicable to states defined by their phenomenology. Crucially this will include pain states within the nursing context. Even a general directive to 'relieve suffering' is answerable to subjective phenomena.

So due to the absence of an epistemic gap between say, being in pain and believing one is in pain, this range of phenomena lacks a crucial realist requirement, this being the presence of ontological depth in a range of phenomena. Bhaskar's conception of realism requires that such depth is present in any range of phenomena amenable to scientific study.

A defence of Bhaskar's position against this criticism may be to argue that the relationship between pain states and neurological states really *is* one such that the former are the appearance of the latter.

But this does not seem promising at all. It does not sound plausible to claim that pain states are less real than neurological structures. And, as Bhaskar allows (since he rejects reductionism) pain cannot be identified with physical states since it is identified by its phenomenology and, as seen in Chapter 5 above, this is not true of any physical state.

More weakly, Bhaskar may argue that the neurological structures are necessary conditions of the possible occurrence of pain. But even if they are necessary conditions of pain, it is hard to envisage how any description or explanation of the function of neurological structures could amount to an explanation of the phenomenon of pain. This is most probably due to the difference in ontological category between pain and any physical phenomenon. So there seem good grounds to reject the realist turn at least as this is set out by Bhaskar.

In summary of the turn to realism: first, the turn to realism draws attention to a possible weakness in interpretivism, specifically that this presupposes realism. An interpretivist can of course accept this; it need only be a fatal objection to a form of interpretivism which rejects realism – such as Benner's interpretive phenomenology.

Second, let us accept that it does indeed provide a satisfactory picture of science. So one condition of adequacy, it appears, is met. But the criticism raised above suggests that acceptance of Bhaskar's realism leads to an incompatibility between nursing and science of the following kind. Bhaskar sets out necessary conditions of any possible object of scientific enquiry. Phenomena of key concern to nursing, it appears, are essentially such that they cannot meet this necessary condition. It follows that nursing cannot be science – that is, on Bhaskar's conception of what science is.

Overall, it seems to me that if the claim that nursing is a science is to be made out, then alignment with some form of interpretivism seems most promising. This does not make the kinds of restrictions on possible objects of scientific enquiry which are made in Bhaskar's view, and is not incompatible with some form of ontological realism.

Problems do remain, however, concerning the extent to which generalisation is possible; and also the possibility that allowing interpretivism to count as science allows in too much else. For example, any activity which includes a role for reason and evidence. Hence on this view even philosophy would count as a science!

Conclusion

It was plain that positivism matches neither a credible conception of nursing nor of science. Bhaskar's realism may well provide a credible conception of science. But, so it was argued here, it does not sit with a credible conception of nursing. This is due to Bhaskar's condition of a possible object of scientific enquiry. That leaves interpretivism. While this is an advance on positivism it remains problematic to claim that nursing is an interpretive science. For as noted, in nursing it is necessarily true that knowledge is sought for instrumental purposes, and this is not true of interpretive science generally. And again, it is necessarily true that nursing has a moral dimension (its intelligibility is dependent upon this), but this is at most contingently present in interpretive science (its intelligibility is not dependent upon its having a moral dimension).

Also, of course, it has to be shown that interpretivism is a credible picture of science. Is this the case? As seen there remains a role for the provision of evidence, within interpretivism. And there is no incompatibility with realism. But there do seem problems. These concern difficulties relating to generalisation, and the problem that an interpretivist conception of science may be overly inclusive. For many activities are compatible with realism, involve interpretation, and assessment of evidence. Stamp collecting, train spotting, and astrology spring to mind for example.

Further, a key objection which can be addressed to each of the three options we discussed is that, as we have seen, they are approaches to knowledge gathering. Acquiring knowledge is of importance to nursing, but as we saw in Chapters 2 and 3 nursing is a practice discipline. Any knowledge acquired, whether by positivist, interpretivist, or realist methodologies – has to be employed (or at least capable of employment). So surely an exclusive focus on these approaches to knowledge acquisition neglects the point that this is a focus merely on *means*. An adequate characterisation must include an account of how relevant knowledge is put into practice to bring about the ends of nursing. Hence, papers such as Wainwright (1997) which is titled 'A new paradigm for nursing: the potential of realism', run the risk of seducing readers into thinking that an improved approach to knowledge gathering will provide a full account of nursing. This is not so.

It is this insight which in part has led to the claim that nursing is an art, or is a combination of art and science. But we will see in the next chapter the view that nursing is an art is vulnerable to strong objection.

Finally, in opposition to the claim that nursing is an applied science it was argued that, strictly speaking, nursing involves the *application* of applied science (see section at the beginning of this chapter). As shown above, engagement in the application of applied science does not make one a scientist (recall the 'bricklayer' example). Moreover, again as argued above, the intelligibility of applied science requires that its objects behave in uniform ways, for example that all samples of a particular chemical substance or plastic have the same properties, and so can be treated in the same way. But no such assumption of 'uniformity' can be made in relation to the nursing care of patients. Pieces of copper all have the same properties and, thus, behave in the same way. Patients do not.

9 *The nature of nursing (ii): nursing as art or practice*

In this chapter we continue our discussion of the nature of nursing. We begin in the first part with the idea of nursing as an art, and then move on in the second part to discuss the view which will be supported here; namely that nursing is most adequately conceived of as a practice.

Nursing as an art

The claim that nursing is an art is also a familiar one within nursing literature (Nightingale, 1957; Chinn and Watson, 1994; Johnson, 1994). Moreover, as we saw earlier (Chapter 3) the situation has been given a further twist by Carper's claim that aesthetics is one of four crucial 'patterns of knowing' in nursing (1978).

In what follows we will adopt a strategy similar to that pursued in our discussion of whether nursing is a science. Hence, as in that discussion, it is a constraint on any answer that what are identified are credible concepts both of nursing and of art. And also, as with the claim that nursing is a science, the claim that nursing is an art is similarly a 'class inclusion' claim. So it is subject to the same constraint on class membership as the claim that nursing is a science. When applied to the claim that nursing is an art, this runs as follows.

It is reasonable to suppose membership of the class of those activities we know as arts hinges upon the possession by those activities of certain key relevant characteristics. It is in virtue of the possession of these characteristics, whatever they are, that certain activities count as art and others do not. Thus, painting, literature and sculpting seem reasonably classed as arts. Biology, botany, and psychology seem not to be. In this section we seek to identify just what characteristics an activity needs to possess in order to ensure inclusion into the class of arts. This will require us to consider one of the most prominent theories of art, that of R.G. Collingwood. Once we do this, it will be evident that nursing lacks the key characteristics of art, as this is understood by Collingwood.

In parallel with points made in the previous discussion of nursing as a science, the fact that nurses use art in their practice does not entail that nursing is an art. In some forms of nursing, say paediatric, or mental health nursing, nurses may use art for broadly therapeutic purposes. Perhaps it is done to help sick children cope with the frustration and boredom of being in hospital; or to encourage people with mental health problems to discuss them – so-called art therapy. It need not follow from this that nursing is, therefore, an art. One may use art to relieve one's boredom but it does not follow from this that relieving boredom is an art.

In parallel with our discussion of science, once again, any attempt to identify nursing with art presupposes some understanding of art. Specifying a straightforward, relatively stable definition of science proved difficult. Providing such a definition of art is at least equally problematic.

Theories of art

However, it is common to distinguish two main accounts of art. According to the first, the imitation (or mimetic) theory, art simply mirrors or attempts to mirror natural phenomena or events in life. This theory derives from Aristotle (for example see his *Poetics*) and Plato (see, for example, *The Republic*). So plays and poems would be mirrors of real lives, paintings copies of real objects or natural phenomena such as landscapes. Music was considered imitative in that it was thought to 'imitate the natural order of the cosmos or the soul' (Gardner, 1995, p. 614).

It should be said at the outset that this does not seem a promising option. The view that the ends of nursing are to mirror natural phenomena could not be part of any credible account of nursing.

The second theory, which emerged in the 19th century, is known as the expressive theory. This posits a necessary relationship between art and the expression of emotion. Here the focus lies not on the object – the work of art itself – but on the artist.

This seems a more promising focus than the mimetic theory in the attempt to define nursing as an art. The presence of certain kinds of mental states are often posited as central to good nursing: for example the presence of a caring attitude (Bishop and Scudder, 1991, p. 53), and the possession of relevant knowledge, are thought crucial to good nursing, and so on.

One of the most well-known expressive theories of art is that proposed by Collingwood (see his *Principles of Art*, 1958). Collingwood (pp. 5–6) points to divergent, historical meanings of the term. In ancient Latin and Greek, for example, the relevant terms (*Ars*, and *techne*) referred generally to any skilled activity. So no distinction was maintained between, say, shoemaking and poetry: each were crafts. Activities which contemporary usage would describe as arts were all covered by the same general term which referred to what would now be termed crafts (carpentry, shoemaking, tailoring and so on).

In medieval Latin *Ars* came to mean simply 'any special form of book-learning' (1958, p. 6) regardless of its subject matter. Then, according to Collingwood, in the late 18th century, a distinction emerged between 'the fine arts and the useful arts' (ibid., p. 6). The former involve much of what we presently regard as art, and the latter much of what we presently regard as craft; so the fine arts include painting, music and literature, and the useful arts include carpentry, shoemaking, tailoring and so on. So according to Collingwood, since roughly the late 18th century, art proper is generally held to be distinct from craft. What is the basis for the distinction?

Collingwood suggests that craft involves 'the power to produce a preconceived result by means of consciously controlled and directed action' (1958, p. 15). Hence, a craftsperson is one who has such power. Thus, a tailor produces a suit as a result of following a design and using appropriate materials and implements in the appropriate fashion.

The main grounds for the art/craft distinction are these:

1. 'Craft always involves a distinction between means and end' (p. 15).

2. Craft 'involves a distinction between planning and executing' (p. 15).

3. In a craft, a craftsman changes the form of some type of matter: for example turns a piece of leather into a shoe; hence, in a craft 'There is a distinction between form and matter' (p. 16).

4. 'There is a hierarchical relation between various crafts' (p. 16). Hence, the craft of the tailor depends upon the craft of the fabric-maker or weaver.

Collingwood, thus, describes medicine as a craft. Its ends are to produce certain states in humans (for example health, freedom from disease), and its means include those which comprise medical knowledge. Similarly, it seems, by Collingwood's understanding of craft, nursing would be categorised as a craft and not an art.

In order to understand more fully the contrast to which Collingwood points it is necessary to consider how he explains why art does not meet the characteristics of craft. For, on the face of it, it may be claimed that a landscape painting, for example, requires a distinction between means and end: the end is the representation of the relevant landscape, the means are the technical skills necessary to execute the representation. Hence condition (1) is met, as is condition (2). Condition (3) is met in that the raw materials of paint and canvas are transformed into a painting; and condition (4) seems met since a similar hierarchy can be pointed to – for example between the painter's 'art' and paintmaking.

However, Collingwood wishes to reject such analyses and to maintain that the landscape artist who proceeds in the way just described does not produce a work of art. For Collingwood, the fact that the 'artist' proceeds in the way described renders his work *craft* and not art. The reason is that Collingwood distinguishes what may be called art from 'art proper'. The landscape painting, thus, is not 'art proper' for him.

There seem close echoes here of much of what is written of the art of nursing (for example, Johnson, 1994). The practice of such art, it is said, does not involve simply following instructions, but involves intuition, care and emotion: aspects of human life which resist step-by-step analysis. 'Art proper', for Collingwood, necessarily involves the imaginative expression of emotion. Hence, the question of whether a work is an example of art or craft is determined entirely by consideration of the process of its production; specifically, the processes which take place within the mind of the artist.

So any kind of activity, the main purpose of which is ends-directed, cannot be art on Collingwood's theory. He identifies a number of types of activity which are essentially ends-directed and which are mistakenly described as art, but which properly speaking are not art but craft. For example, he identifies representative art, what he terms 'magical art', and 'amusement art', none of which count as art proper. The reasons why stem from the fact that these kinds of 'art' are ends-directed.

Consider, for example, representative art. If the main purpose of this is to mirror or imitate part of reality as closely as possible – perhaps a portrait of a person, or a favourite landscape – it cannot count as art. For the end is that of faithful representation and this, simply, is not an 'artistic end' (1958, p. 45) for Collingwood, and is simply a technical skill.

With reference to 'magical art', this is said to encompass religious and patriotic art; that is, it is art aimed at bringing about a specific practical end (ibid., p. 69). For example, the production of religious awe, or patriotic feelings in an audience. Hence this does not count as art proper for Collingwood in that it is primarily produced for ends which are only contingently of concern to the artist. The primary end of such works is the production of an effect in the audience, and not with the expression of the artist's emotion.

As might be anticipated, 'amusement art' does not qualify as art proper; its primary purpose is the entertainment of the audience, and this, in art proper, is irrelevant. Hence much popular music would not count as art. Examples of amusement art given by Collingwood include thriller writing and pornography (1958, pp. 84–5). Overall then, any activity which is primarily ends-related cannot count as art proper for Collingwood.

As we have heard, for him, art proper essentially involves the expression of emotion. This is not to say that the mere expression of emotion equals art. Neither a wail of sorrow, nor a cry of fear count as works of art. The reason is that emotions expressed in this way are not considered by Collingwood to be under the control of the person. It appears necessary that some kind of reflection and control of the emotion is required. This makes it possible for the emotion to be expressed properly. As he puts it:

> The characteristic mark of expression proper is lucidity or intelligibility; a person who expresses something thereby becomes conscious of what it is that he is expressing, and enables others to become conscious of it in himself and in them (1958, p. 122).

So, plausibly, it is held that the mere expression of emotion does not itself amount to art. It has to be expressed in some kind of symbolic fashion, for example in words, or on canvas, or in music.

Given this qualification, Collingwood suggests the proposal that art essentially involves the expression of emotion is one which is commonplace; it is one 'familiar to every artist, and to everyone else who has any acquaintance with the arts' (1958, p. 109). Further, Collingwood suggests that artistic expressions of emotion are primarily for the artist themselves; it is a matter of making clear to oneself how one is feeling or how one felt, and giving expression to this in some symbolic form.

The generation of a work of art is said to involve an act of creation on the part of the artist, and it is one which essentially employs imagination. Thus the artist must have both unexpressed emotion within her, and have the imagination to express this in symbolic fashion.

Conceived of in this way, then, art in contrast to craft, is said not to involve a specified end which is then obtained by specified means. Rather, there is no discernible end. In art proper, the art simply emerges from the imaginative expression of emotion. The final work is not planned and then executed; rather it emerges from the creative process.

Some considerations in support of Collingwood's account include the following: the theory is able to account for the intuition that a photograph of a person does not amount to a work of art: it's a mere 'copy' of reality. Painting a picture which so closely resembles a person, say, that it represents them as closely as a photograph clearly requires a great deal of skill. But this is simply like the skill of the draughtsman or carpenter: that is, it is a craft. The same applies to fake art: that is, the copying of original works. Also, by Collingwood's criterion, computer-generated 'art' would not constitute art proper. For, although a representation might be excellent, the product would not derive from expressed emotion, nor presumably from imagination. Further, in relation to the performance of music, Collingwood's account lends support to the view that improvised passages in music constitute art in that they involve the expression of emotion. This is in contrast with simply following a pre-ordained sequence of notes; this latter would not constitute art by Collingwood's thesis.

Hence the differences between art and craft can be summarised as follows:

1. Whereas craft always requires a means/end distinction, art does not. The reason is that the end is not clear to the artist until it is produced. So there is no preconceived end.

2. Relatedly, whereas craft involves a distinction between planning and executing, these are not separable in art. Any 'plan' would be the work of art itself. For example, consider the production of a short poem. One might mentally try out different verses before one ended up with a final

version – all in one's head. There is no equivalent of the planning and executing phases here.

3. In craft there is a transformation of one kind of material into another. Collingwood (1958, pp. 22–3) denies that words can be regarded as 'material' suitably transformed into a poem. Similarly, he denies that this could be said of emotion. So it is held that there is no raw material which is transformed into a final product.

4. Finally, the hierarchical relations between crafts is not present in arts. Although Collingwood allows that poetry may be set to music he denies that this constitutes a hierarchy. Part of the reason being that the poem can stand alone as a work of art independently of its recruitment by the musician. Craft materials, however, are produced specifically for recruitment by others (for example the leather is produced by the tanner for the use of others).

Comments

It was mentioned earlier, then, that nursing cannot be an art by Collingwood's criterion, it can only be classified as a craft.

On a different matter, Collingwood's work draws attention to the significance of the phenomena of emotion and imagination. It seems plain that these are central to good nursing. Witnessing suffering provokes proper emotional responses in nurses, and others of course, and prompts interventions on the part of the nurse to prevent further suffering. Imagination also seems to have a central role in nursing. It requires imagination to anticipate and to meet adequately the needs of patients and their relatives (see Scott, 2000). It may be thought that since emotion and imagination are so central to nursing, and so central to Collingwood's theory that the claims of nursing to be an art can be salvaged.

However, this does not seem likely. The reason is that as we have seen, Collingwood's theory places the artist at the centre of matters. It is the emotions of the artist which are of primary importance. And similarly, it is the imaginative work which the artist performs upon his own mental experiences which is crucial. In short, being primarily other-regarding rather than self-regarding is central to nursing; the position is the opposite of that proposed by Collingwood.

Are we to suppose, then, that nursing is a craft? There are some similarities between Collingwood's description of crafts and nursing. As we have seen, it does seem possible to distinguish means and ends within nursing. And specific nursing actions can also be considered as means to ends, for example taking a patient's temperature.

It is fair to say that the notion of a craft seems too 'thin' to adequately characterise nursing. The kinds of phenomena mentioned in our discussion of the unsuitability of positivism are significant here. Suppose we take wheelbuilding as a typical example of a craft and compare it to nursing. It involves dexterity and skilled manipulation of materials, and we may reasonably suppose nursing to require this also, in some clinical contexts at least. But there is no necessary moral dimension to crafts, yet there is to nursing. And of course the objects with which the craftsperson is concerned do not have subjectivity – wheels do not have mental experiences – so a layer of interpretive complexity which is present in nursing is wholly absent in crafts. Think also of our discussion of care. There it was seen that the intelligibility of nursing rests upon its being a response to human vulnerability. But the idea of vulnerability seems not to be central to crafts. Rather like the applied scientist, the craftsperson relies upon the materials she works with having the same properties. There is no requirement to treat individual samples of a kind any differently; nor could there be any rationale for this. Yet our discussions on care and the person show that patients do require such individual consideration. So, as with applied science, it seems a necessary feature of crafts that the objects worked on – for example spokes, rims and so on – each have the same properties (that each spoke made of the same material will be capable of bearing the same amount of weight for example). As we saw, this is not the case in nursing. Here there is a requirement to treat individual 'samples' of a kind differently and not to assume they are the same. These considerations count strongly against the conception of nursing as a mere craft.

Of course it may be said that the idea of art appealed to in the claim that nursing is an art is really the claim that nursing involves the skilled performance of an activity. In this way it is analogous to the art of the wheelbuilder or tailor. But this sounds simply like the claim that nursing is a craft. As just explained wheelbuilding and activities like it are more properly viewed as crafts. And this is too thin a concept to do justice to nursing. It masks the interpretive and moral complexity of nursing practice. There is no equivalent to these layers of complexity within either art or crafts.

I have omitted to discuss a 'combined view' which is sometimes mentioned to the effect that nursing is an art and a science. But of course if the idea of nursing as an art is inadequate, and so too is the idea of nursing as a science, there seems no reason to expect the combined view will be successful. Neither of these concepts does justice to the layers of complexity present within nursing at the levels of morals, interpretation, sensitivity to the vulnerability of others, and practical knowledge.

It is, perhaps, in the light of considerations such as this, and dissatisfaction with the construal of nursing as a science, that a third claim has emerged. This is the view that nursing is a *practice* (see Bishop and Scudder, 1991, 1997; P. Wainwright, 1997; Sellman, 2000).

Nursing as a practice

Our discussion of nursing as art concluded with the view that although it is unlikely that nursing is an art, it may be a craft. But brief analysis of this option suggests that this is too 'thin' a concept with which to identify nursing. Nursing is such a rich area of activity within which morals, interpretation, and grasp of subjectivity are crucial, in addition to the performance of practical skills. While the idea of a craft might help to capture what is involved in the latter, it cannot hope to encompass the former three central elements of nursing. And as noted, the idea of nursing as a combination of art and science is also inadequate.

In recent years the idea that nursing is a practice has been presented as a third possibility. Notable proponents of this idea are Bishop and Scudder (1991, 1997, 1999), among others. They argue that the most legitimate method to try to identify the nature of nursing is to conduct a 'phenomenological interpretation of nursing' (1991, p. 6). This involves focusing on the 'lived experience of the practice of nursing' (p. 6). The adequacy of any account which emerges from such a phenomenological interpretation is to be tested against their readers own experiences of nursing. Bishop and Scudder are, of course, confident that when this is done their own analysis will be supported.

Their strategy contrasts with approaches which are motivated by other, non-practice led considerations. For example, in considering the claim that nursing is a science, it was noted that one motivation for this is to capture some of the status of science by describing nursing as a science. This may then lead to the attempt to 'warp' nursing practice to fit in with the conception of science held by those who favour such a project. Clearly such a process involves an attempt to impose a particular view of 'how nursing should be' upon nursing as currently practised. Moreover, it is an attempt to change nursing 'from without' so to speak, by importing into nursing elements of another area of activity, in this case science. In contrast to such approaches, Bishop and Scudder's strategy is to commence with practice as it currently is.

Their attempt to do this involves focusing on some 'exemplars of nursing excellence' (1991, p. 15), many of which are drawn from Benner's work (1984). Focusing on these examples, leads them to claim that nursing is, in fact, a *caring practice* (p. 95, and *passim*). Briefly, their proposal is that the instances of nursing excellence which they describe reveal nursing to involve caring for others. We saw in Chapter 8 that this is a plausible claim, although not one which distinguishes nursing from other 'caring practices' such as parenting, social work and so on in that it points to necessary but not sufficient conditions of nursing.

In order to explicate fully what the claim that nursing is a practice amounts to, we will focus on the idea of a practice as this is set out by MacIntyre. As with the claims that nursing is a science or an art, the claim that nursing is a practice is also a class inclusion claim. In order to assess the proposal that nursing is a practice we need to gain an idea of the types of characteristics that are necessary for membership of the class of practices.

In a trivial sense, nursing is something which is practised. Again trivially, one cannot be a nurse unless one knows how to practise; and as suggested in our discussion of practical knowing (Chapter 2), this knowledge itself can be obtained only by engaging in practice. But a more interesting, richer, sense of practice is one which MacIntyre describes as follows. He writes:

> By a 'practice' I am going to mean any coherent and complex form of socially estab-lished cooperative human activity through which goods internal to that form of activity are realized in the course of trying to achieve those standards of excellence which are appropriate to, and partially definitive of, that form of social activity, with the result that human powers to achieve excellence, and human conceptions of ends and goods involved are systematically extended (1985, p. 187).

As examples of practices MacIntyre lists football, chess, architecture, farming, physics, history and music, among others (ibid., p. 187). Let us go through MacIntyre's definition more slowly in order to try to be clear about how the claim that *nursing* is a practice in this sense can be understood.

A key distinction which is central to MacIntyre's notion is that between internal and external goods. He uses the example of an adult teaching a child how to play chess. At first the adult might reward the child with sweets to coax him to persisting with learning the game. So in the early phases of learning the game, the game itself is of only instrumental value from the child's point of view: it is a means towards the end of gaining rewards such as sweets.

But gradually as the child begins to learn how to play, and discovers the pleasures of playing chess, the child comes to want to play the game for its own sake. In MacIntyre's terms, this is the stage at which the child discovers the goods which are *internal* to playing chess. Such goods 'cannot be had in any way but by playing chess or some game of that specific kind' (ibid., p. 188). Such goods can be contrasted with external goods, which of course in MacIntyre's example of the chess-playing child, are the sweets. These *can* be obtained in ways other than by participating in a practice.

In addition to being available only by participation in a practice, internal goods, it is claimed, 'can only be identified and recognized by the experience of participating in the practice in question' (1985, pp. 188–9). So in relation to chess, it would follow, first, that the goods internal to this are only avail-able by playing chess. And second, one can only recognise the goods internal to chess if one has experience of playing chess.

Let us apply some of this to nursing, then. Take the first part of MacIn-tyre's definition (the first four lines of the above quoted passage). It is reason-able to describe nursing as a 'coherent and complex form of... human activity' (ibid.). Its coherence is evident from works such as Benner 1984, and Benner and Wrubel, 1989; in these texts examples are given of 'good nursing'.

(Though some care is needed here since, as noted, what constitutes good practice is not fixed for all time, so to speak. As will be seen below, this can be viewed as a positive feature of practices; unchanging practices become ossified.) And there are education and training courses with established concerns and syllabuses. So the coherence of nursing can be noted. With regard to its complexity, our discussions of knowledge, persons and care as these bear upon nursing point to this. So claims of coherence and complexity seem sustainable.

Still focusing on the early part of the definition we find a reference to internal goods. These, it is claimed, 'are realized in the course of trying to achieve those standards of excellence...[and so on]' One way to construe the idea of internal goods here is as those goods which are manifested in excellent nursing practice.

Our previous discussions of knowledge, persons and care drew attention to three areas within nursing which any account of nursing must encompass – that is, relating to knowledge, persons and, via care, its moral dimension. With a view to showing that these dimensions can be incorporated within the conception of nursing as a practice, let us try to consider them in terms of internal goods.

First, with reference to knowledge, mastery of the technical dimension of nursing can be mentioned here. The dexterity involved in using medical equipment, sphygmomanometers, ampoules, syringes, needles and drips, is important to many areas of hospital-based nursing. As with the other two dimensions mentioned, skill in this dimension comes with experience, with acculturation into the practice of nursing. It cannot be gathered without performing the tasks. Further, given what was said in our discussion of practical knowing, it is likely that even this kind of practical knowing cannot be obtained outside the practice setting. For it is one thing to practise drawing up a drug into a syringe in the classroom and a wholly different thing to do this on the ward setting, with the patient there, or with other nurses close by. One knows they will detect any signs of hesitation, nervousness, or lack of dexterity.

Second, our account of the person shows that considerable interpretive skill is required of the nurse. Good nursing requires the acquisition of a sense of the patient's construal of his symptoms. A good nurse can be expected to possess such skills and to manifest these in her work. Partly in virtue of the possession of such skills, such a nurse would be regarded as a good nurse. Such skills do not come readily and have to be learned over time during practice. It is such skills which, in Benner's terms, help partially to define the expert nurse. For interpretive judgements derive from experience of numerous situations in past practice, and lead to the formation of the skills in 'pattern recognition' which she describes. Thus interpretive skills are necessary not only in respect of interpreting the deliberate acts and speech of patients, but in the interpretation of their physical condition also (cf. Chapter 4 above).

Hence such interpretive skills can also be cast in terms of internal goods in the construal of nursing as a practice.

Lastly, it is reasonable to suppose internal goods will include *moral* goods, since as we have observed, nursing has an intrinsically moral aspect. Thus at least one class of goods which are internal goods will be moral. We can envisage that these will involve the kind of virtues which one would hope a nurse possesses, for example respect for others, compassion, care, empathy, honesty, integrity, courage, a sense of justice, and so on. Thus, instances of good nursing are likely to involve one or more of these moral characteristics.

Relatedly, Bishop and Scudder report on a sense of fulfilment which many nurses experience after an episode in which they feel they nursed a patient especially well. In the example they give, a nurse writes of 'the joy obtained by providing emotional and physical support' (1991, p. 25) to a dying patient and her family. Although perhaps 'joy' is the wrong word, Bishop and Scudder point to the sense of fulfilment which the nurse experienced as a result of the way she nursed this patient.

So, then, we have discussed three kinds of internal goods (relating to knowledge, persons and the moral dimension of nursing care) which on the face of it are central to nursing.

Still focusing on the early part of MacIntyre's definition, note that the goods internal to nursing arise in the course of trying to practise good nursing (at least this is a reasonable reading of the first lines of the above quote). Thus it is reasonable to conclude they feature among the means by which the ends of nursing are achieved. In a nurse's ordinary day-to-day practice, on this view, the nurse is trying to be a good nurse, in other words, is trying to meet the 'standards of excellence' appropriate to nursing.

In the last three lines of the quote it is suggested that the relevant standards of excellence are 'partially definitive' of the practice. Thus in nursing, exemplars of good nursing, reasonably enough, would be taken to partially define nursing. So if one was asked, 'What is nursing?' one could point to an exemplar of good nursing. As we heard, this is precisely the strategy adopted by Bishop and Scudder. In trying to characterise nursing, one focuses on exemplars of good practice.

We noted earlier two features of internal goods on MacIntyre's view. According to the first feature the goods internal to a practice are only available by engaging in that practice. So, acceptance of the claim that nursing is a practice, requires acceptance of the view that there is such a class of goods. I would suppose that medicine is the activity which most closely approximates nursing, in terms of internal goods. Medicine, too, involves moral, interpretive and technical dimensions. But a key difference, often pointed to, between nursing and medicine concerns the nature of the relationship with patients in the two domains. It is common to observe that nurses have more contact with patients than doctors; and that nurses often 'translate' the information given by doctors to patients for them. Bishop and Scudder suggest that nurses are in an 'in-between' position (1991, p. 18); that is, nurses occupy the territory between doctors and patients. So although there are close similarities between nursing and medicine, important differences can be pointed to.

Remaining with this first feature of internal goods, it may be claimed that the goods internal to nursing are also present in, say, parenthood. But against this, surely the relationship between a parent and a child is importantly different from that between a nurse and a patient. The nurse is in a professional relationship with the patient, and this is likely to be a temporary relationship. This is not the case (typically) with parent–child relations.

So the first feature of internal goods seems to stand up to scrutiny, and to being placed within the nursing context. What of the second, that is, that internal goods can only be recognised by those who have participated in the relevant practice. This too seems a reasonable claim. Let us suppose that novice nurses count as people who have not yet participated in the practice of nursing; they are in the very early stages of their education. It is reasonable to suppose they may not recognise exemplars of good nursing as such until this is pointed out to them, and the reasons why explained.

As a crude example, suppose a novice nurse visits an acute care unit in the mental health context and sees a nurse playing scrabble with a patient. The novice's impression is that this has nothing to do with good nursing, and more to do with the laziness of the nurse. The nurse then explains that the patient had previously been very withdrawn and that playing this quiet game represents a major step forward for the patient. Moreover, the nurse has ensured that the game takes place in a specific part of the unit, one from where most of the unit is visible. Thus the nurse explains to the novice her practice. It is reasonable to suppose this is evident only to those who have experience of nursing in this kind of context.

Note too that this example shows how internal goods resist 'parcelling up', defining in terms of inputs and outputs. To those outside the practice, the nurse is playing scrabble with a patient. This description omits to take into account the degree of prior contact – say, apparently minor contact such as a glance, or a smile – which had occurred between the nurse and the patient for days prior to the game. Assuming participation in the game is indeed of benefit to the patient, how could the occurrence of the game be properly described in terms of inputs and outputs? When would the inputs begin and end? Would a glance count as an input? Can the degree of well-being which is the output of the game be quantified? It seems absurd to suppose it could.

A clear implication of this view appears to be that those who have no knowledge of nursing cannot undertake assessment of nursing practice. (We discuss a problem with this shortly.)

Bishop and Scudder point to a further important implication of considering nursing as a practice. Suppose it is accepted that the ends of nursing are of the kind we have mentioned previously, relieving suffering, promoting well-being and so on. On the view of practices so far set out, the goods internal to the practice must be bound to these ends. They are goods in so far as they make it the case that these ends are brought about. So even tasks such as keeping a linen cupboard tidy, and doing administrative work owe their sense due to their relation, ultimately, with the ends of nursing. At some level the legitimacy of nurses undertaking such activities must connect up with their having a relationship to the ends of nursing, of making it more rather than less likely that the ends of nursing can be met. So if keeping the linen cupboard tidy or the performance of administrative tasks do not ultimately connect up with the ends of nursing, there is no place for them within nursing. Thus a nurse who undertakes administrative work for its own sake, or to realise goods external to nursing – for example higher pay – cannot be said to be participating in the practice of nursing. Such a person 'ceases being a nurse and becomes a bureaucrat' (Bishop and Scudder, 1991, p. 34).

And finally, in exposition of MacIntyre's definition, the last three lines of it involve the claim that our conceptions of ends will be enriched and, thus, extended. Hence pursuance of the internal goods of nursing may be said to generate a richer conception of human ends and goods. This may involve a richer understanding of nursing work and the ends it seeks to bring about, for example, a more adequate understanding of suffering and how to relieve it, a more adequate account of the moral dimension in nursing, and a more adequate account of the place for interpretation in nursing. It is plausible to claim that there have been significant developments in each of these areas within the last few decades.

Having set out the rudiments of the conception of nursing as a practice, we turn to consider some concerns which can be raised against it.

Criticisms

A first criticism stems from the claim that only those within a practice can recognise the goods internal to it (MacIntyre, 1985, pp. 188–9). This may be interpreted as a claim that only those within a practice can recognise good practice. Obvious grounds for concern here arise in relation to mental health nursing, and nursing people with serious intellectual disabilities. Over the past thirty years in the UK it has emerged that patients in institutions for the care of such people were often seriously abused. It seems reasonable to point out that were people from outside the practice of nursing brought in to witness such abuse taking place, they could easily have recognised it as abuse. For example, it is hard to imagine any plausibly therapeutic grounds for kicking a patient. Yet this is the kind of aggression that patients were being subjected to.

In partial defence of MacIntyre's line here, the definition itself as stated above restricts its claim to what constitutes *good* practice, not what constitutes bad. In the quoted passage there is no claim that bad practice cannot be recognised by 'outsiders', only that good practice cannot. This seems a much more plausible claim.

For example, suppose a nurse spends a great deal of time with one particular patient, at the expense of her responsibilities to others. While that patient may judge the nurse to be a good nurse, other nurses seem best placed to make a proper evaluation. Their view may be that the nurse's performance does not meet appropriate standards due to her neglect of other patients. Of course it may be said that other patients can point this out perfectly well. But in some circumstances it may be that a nurse *is* justified in spending more time with one patient, even if at the expense of others, if there are good grounds to do so. Such grounds must be ones which connect up with the goods internal to nursing. For example, it may be that the nurse judges that a particular patient with a history of schizophrenia is on the very edge of breaking down, of having a relapse. Thus the nurse may judge it appropriate to spend more time with that patient at the risk of neglecting others. In such circumstances it seems reasonable to suppose that other nurses are better placed than that nurse's patients to judge whether the nurse's practice is sound or otherwise.

A second concern is that the MacIntyrean line simply entrenches the status quo. (Recall also here the charge of conservatism levelled at Benner in Chapter 3.) Defining good nursing by what is currently regarded as good nursing surely obstructs any new ideas, new and possibly better ways of doing things. To see the force of this worry one need only recall what used to be considered 'good nursing' in the mid part of the 20th century. This involved the regimentation of patients' routines, and an obsession with order (beds in a perfect line, perfectly made, linen cupboards stacked in perfect geometric order, and so on). In the mental health context it was considered more important to make beds than to talk to patients. This is a worry evident in Bishop and Scudder's 'phenomenological' method which boils down to a strategy of defining nursing by reference to that which is currently regarded as good nursing.

In defence of the MacIntyrean position, his conception of a practice is such that it is a 'continuous argument' (1985, p. 222). In other words within the practice there is continuous discussion and debate concerning the nature of the practice, for example of its ends, of the means necessary to meet them, of how the practice is best taught to novices, and so on.

It should be said that this conception of practice sits well with the view of knowledge favoured in Chapter 2 above. There it was claimed that we should regard our knowledge claims with an attitude of modesty. We should be open to the possibility that our currently favoured views are in need of revision; and of the possibility that the evidence we recruit in favour of currently favoured views does not give a fair chance to rival views.

Thus the idea of *criticism* is central to the idea of a practice. Moreover, it has been suggested in the present work that such questioning of the basic nature of a practice is characteristic of philosophical enquiry. So the conception of nursing as a practice may even help to articulate further the importance of philosophy of nursing to nursing. For the presence of philosophical questioning, especially from those within the practice, can contribute to the further development and extension of nursing considered as a practice.

A third concern involves the distinction between internal and external goods. Surely, these are not wholly separable. For in order to practise nursing one has to have *some* external goods in order to be fit to practise. One needs food and housing, and in fact a reasonable standard of living.

Once more, however, there is a defence available to MacIntyre. This is to suggest that the relationship between internal and external goods need not be one in which they are essentially separable. It remains possible to maintain that the two types of goods are distinct, but that in order to be in a position to experience internal goods, one needs external goods. This relationship is parallel to something like that between needing oxygen and acting morally. One needs oxygen in order to be capable of so acting, but we can still distinguish oxygen and moral actions.

Before closing this discussion of nursing conceived of as a practice, it is important to draw attention to a serious weakness in Bishop and Scudder's discussion. As mentioned earlier, they present the idea of a practice as a third alternative to the idea that nursing is a science or an art. (See their paper 'Nursing as a practice...' (1997).)

But clearly, at least given MacIntyre's definition, science and art could equally be construed as practices – indeed, physics is one of his own examples of a practice (1985, p. 187). In science we can think of internal goods such as the intellectual virtues of diligence, the dogged pursuance of a problem, the employment of analytical and imaginative skills, and so on. External goods, are the same as with other practices – fame, riches, and so on. So if it is accepted that nursing is a practice, this in itself is not sufficient to establish that it is neither a science, nor an art.

However, suppose it is accepted that science and art do constitute practices in MacIntyre's sense, it does still seem possible to distinguish nursing from science and from art. As discussed in the previous chapter, nursing seems importantly different from science. Nursing practice is inseparable from a concern with human vulnerability, well-being and suffering, its very intelligibility is inseparable from its moral dimension. This seems not to be the case with science (in the modern sense). Its essential characteristic is that of knowledge seeking. The intrinsic aim of science is to obtain knowledge about the world. Whether or not this has instrumental value is an entirely contingent matter.

But, as we saw, with nursing any knowledge gathering which does take place – and thus any science which is undertaken within nursing practice – is, of *necessity*, primarily of instrumental value only. Its use is subservient to the ends of nursing, making people well, relieving pain and suffering and so on. So even where nursing involves the application of science, nothing follows from this to the effect that nursing is a science.

It may be claimed that nursing can be applied in a 'scientific way' – and hence is an applied science. Thus, it may be claimed, nursing may be assimilated to practices such as engineering (for example building bridges or buildings). But as we saw in our discussion of realism and positivism a crucial difference between nursing and such activities is that nursing practice is answerable to subjective considerations in ways in which engineering, say, is not. There are objective criteria which can be employed to determine whether or not the ends of engineering have been met – does the bridge function properly? does the building stay up? and so on. And more obviously, nursing is concerned with beings with subjectivity (this is a necessary truth about nursing), applied science cannot be (that is, given the necessity to treat samples of the same kinds of materials as equivalent).

Our considerations in relation to the view that nursing is an art showed this to be an unlikely claim, given a reasonable view of how the term art should be understood.

Given the problematic nature of claims that nursing is a science, or an art, we can set aside the claim that it is a combination of these. This suggestion serves only to generate further confusion in my view.

Conclusion

With reference to our three candidate terms to capture the nature of nursing, any adequate account of nursing must be rich enough to encompass its complexity. So an adequate account of nursing must have a place to accommodate our conclusions in epistemology, ontology and morality. As seen, these include the revisability of knowledge; the ontological claims regarding persons; and the idea of nursing as a moral response to human vulnerability.

The closest contender for such a general concept looks like that of a practice. It seems a rich enough concept to be compatible with a credible account of nursing. The defining features of a practice, as we saw after our discussion, can be shown to sit well with nursing. Although the idea that a practice is a continuous argument sits more comfortably with nursing in recent years than in previous years, the intrusion of philosophy can be taken as an encouraging sign to try to address this. And, as Cash (1998) has pointed out, certain moral values do seem to have endured throughout the history of nursing.

Those who have a special enthusiasm for the conception of nursing as a science may attempt to characterise nursing as a *scientific* practice. But given the problems we had in sustaining the claim that nursing is a science, this does not seem a promising move. Perhaps the best hope for the conception of nursing as a scientific practice is to try to rehabilitate the ancient sense of that term. But, it must be asked, why do this? Surely this merely generates further confusion as to the nature of nursing. Those who see nursing described as a science will interpret that to mean it is a science in the modern sense. Why proliferate that (mis)conception?

The idea of a practice seems rich enough to embrace features crucial to the ends of nursing such as moral sensitivity, and features central to the means, such as interpretive, theoretical and practical skill. And if construed as a practice in which there is a critical tradition, the articulation of nursing as a practice can be pursued further (again see P. Wainwright, 1997; Cash, 1998; Sellman, 2000).

If nursing is, then, to be conceived of as a practice, it seems reasonable to require that the relations between the means and ends of nursing be understood, or are such that they are at least capable of being rendered coherent. This seems a plausible requirement for the 'unity' of practices as these are described by MacIntyre.

The connecting up of means and ends in nursing is attempted by the provision of nursing theories. But a key feature of nursing as described in Chapters 6 and 7 is its focus on the individual patient. Does this, then, entail that the relations between means and ends cannot be rationalised? Such a 'rationalisation' surely requires generalisations relating means and ends. But the 'individual' nature of nursing seems evident from our discussions of narrative identity and identity-constituting care.

So we have a tension: articulation of nursing as a coherent practice requires the connecting up of means and ends. Yet the 'individual' nature of nursing, generated by our discussions of narrative and the relations of this to health and so on, seems to exclude the possibility of the kinds of generalisations necessary for the articulation of the relations between means and ends. This, in turn, seems to jeopardise the coherence of nursing understood as a practice (and needless to add, as a science).

Yet it is plain that generalisations at some level are relevant to nursing (most obviously, those relating to the biological make-up of humans). But such generalisations must connect up at some point to the achievement of the ends of nursing (otherwise why consider such generalisations relevant?). The attempt to characterise these relations between the means and ends of nursing amounts to the attempt to provide a theory of nursing. As noted, the role of such a theory is to relate means and ends. But our deliberations within the present text seem to threaten this whole project. For, as we heard, although patients may be biologically equivalent – equivalent in terms of biological understanding – it does not follow from this they are equivalent in terms of narrative understanding. Our deliberations so far suggest this latter kind of understanding is the more important of the two, since the purpose of biological understanding is solely instrumental (as our discussion of the nature of scientific enquiry shows). The particular, individual nature of narrative understanding seems to militate against the possibility of generalisations at the level of interactions between nurses and patients. In order to pursue this central ambiguity further we consider the idea of a theory of nursing in our final chapter.

SUGGESTIONS FOR FURTHER READING

Science

Quine and Ullian (1978) as mentioned earlier, is a useful and accessible introduction to philosophy of science. So too is Chalmers (1999). Bhaskar's work, discussed within Chapter 8 is difficult reading, although very important (1975, 1989). Fay (1996) is a useful, clear introduction to philosophy of social science.

The edited collection by Polifroni and Welch (1999) is an excellent source of original articles on the topic of nursing science, and more generally on the topic of philosophy of science as this bears upon nursing.

Art

The Collingwood text discussed in the chapter is accessible and a good read. Dickie (1971) gives an accessible discussion of the subject matter of aesthetics in his *Aesthetics, An Introduction* (Indianapolis: Pegasus); so too does the Gardner paper (1995) referred to in the text. See also O. Hanfling (1992) (ed.) *Philosophical Aesthetics, An Introduction*, Oxford: Oxford University Press. The Chinn and Watson (1994) edited volume gives a useful indication of the way in which claims that nursing is an art or has an aesthetics can be developed. See also the papers by de Raeve (1998) and Wainwright (1999) on this topic.

Practice

As mentioned, the idea that nursing may be a practice in MacIntyre's sense exploits MacIntyre (1985), which is fascinating and accessible. The idea is developed fully in P. Wainwright (1997), and also, in Bishop and Scudder (1991). Sellman (2000) also provides a clear, critical account of the proposal. Dunne (1993) provides the most thorough, careful modern treatment of the idea of a practice, as far as I am aware.

10 The prospects for a theory of nursing

In this chapter an attempt is made to show that the view of the person outlined in Chapters 5 and 7 need not jeopardise the prospects for the articulation of nursing as a practice. It will be argued here that the 'unity' requirement on practices can be sustained. This is achieved by the presentation of a defence of the idea of a theory of nursing. Although no such specific theory is attempted, strategies to overcome apparent obstacles to the development of a theory are set out.

Following a preamble on the concept of theory, we move on to consider the work of Dickoff and James (1968) in relation to the development of nursing theory. Next we see how the generalisations necessary for theory can be compatible with a narrative view of the person. We then describe and deal with two further obstacles to the articulation of a nursing theory. As will be seen, our conclusions will not jeopardise the prospects for the articulation of a theory of nursing.

Preamble

As mentioned, in this final chapter we look more closely at the programme to develop a theory of nursing. It is a programme which has been pursued with considerable vigour over the past four decades (see King and Fawcett, 1997).

As seen in our discussion of nursing as a practice, the kind of relating of means and ends characteristic of theories of nursing seems an important aspect of a unified practice. If the articulation of such a theory proves possible (one which respects key aspects of nursing practice such as those proposed in our discussion so far) it will contribute further to the articulation of nursing as a practice. An apparent obstacle to the development of any such theory stems from the tension, noted on several occasions so far, between the attempt to provide the kind of generalisations apparently required for a nursing theory, and the attempt to individualise care.

It is worth pausing briefly here to consider why it has been thought important to develop such a theory. Presumably, the answer to this is that it is thought that a theory provides a rationalised *systematic* approach to nursing work. This is plainly preferable to an essentially *arbitrary* way of caring for patients. Also, the hope is that in addition to being systematic, the theory will bring about better care for patients. A theory would also be of educational value; novices could learn it. And as noted, a nursing theory would contribute to the further articulation of nursing as a coherent, unified *practice*.

With reference to theories in general, it is standardly claimed they provide explanations, involve descriptions, and enable predictions to be made. And it is possible to identify three minimal constraints which a theory would need to satisfy. Thus suppose someone claims to have developed a theory of asthma:

1. A first requirement would be a description of the phenomena to be explained. In the case of asthma this would be a description of the signs and symptoms of asthma, for example wheezing, shortness of breath and so on (manifest phenomena to use Bhaskar's terms).

2. The proposer would need to be able to identify a single cause or a group of causes of the occurrence of asthma. More strictly speaking, the proposer would need to specify a restricted set of conditions which, when realised, lead to the development of asthma in an individual. Thus suppose the proposer identified conditions A, B, and C such that when these are realised they jointly cause asthma in an individual.

3. An account would be required of the mechanisms which relate the presence of A–C in an individual with the development of asthma, for example how they are responsible for the development of that condition within an individual.

It is reasonable to suppose that the three types of conditions A–C would specify states within an individual (for example genetic structure, or structures within the respiratory system of the individual), and also states beyond an individual (for example environmental irritants).

Let us leave open the precise modality of the relationship between our conditions A–C and the development of asthma. Thus the relations between the occurrence of A–C and the development of asthma could range from necessary relations such that A–C necessarily cause asthma, to (the more likely option) relations of some specified probability (for example in 8 cases out of 10).

I take it that for this to constitute a *theory* of asthma, it would be expected to be generalisable to other humans. It would not count as a theory if it could apply only to one person. (Recall Quine and Ullian's 'virtues'; and see also Chalmers, 1990 on the striving for generality in science.)

To count as a theory of asthma it must be possible to test the theory. This, presumably, would involve looking at other people with asthma to confirm (or falsify) the claim that their asthma is due to their exposure to conditions A–C. And of course efforts would have to be made to try to establish that it is in fact conditions A–C which lead to asthma, and not some other set of conditions D–F which coincidentally accompany conditions A–C.

Even given this overly simple sketch of what is involved in a theory it is evident how a theory can be said to provide explanations, generate predictions, and to rest upon descriptions.

The theory provides an explanation of asthma by identifying the causes of it (that is, conditions A–C and so on) together with a description of its signs and symptoms (wheezing, shortness of breath and so on). So our understanding of asthma is now increased. This in turn enables the generation of predictions such that if an individual is exposed to conditions A–C then he will (or is likely to) develop asthma. Descriptions are of course involved both in the specification of the condition itself, the specification of the conditions A–C, and the mechanisms which link the instancing in an individual of A–C with the signs and symptoms of the condition (for example the mechanism by which cold air brings on the symptoms of asthma).

A similar story could be given in relation to theories of, say, tidal movement or cot death/sudden infant death syndrome. Theories of such phenomena specify the phenomena to be explained by descriptions, then seek to identify conditions which bring about instances of the phenomena, and the mechanisms connecting the relevant conditions with the phenomena to be explained. Such theories require generalisations, must be subjected to testing, and be capable of generating predictions.

With these general remarks on theory in mind let us now look at a landmark paper on the topic of a theory of nursing. The authors note that any such theory must meet the conditions which must be satisfied by all theories, and so they seek to set these out.

Dickoff and James on theory

According to Dickoff and James 'a theory is a conceptual system or framework invented to some purpose' (1968, p. 198). This definition coheres with what has just been claimed. The purpose of natural science is to describe how the world is constituted, and how parts of it are related and so on. And theories in this domain can be expected to generate predictions and so on which either confirm or call into question the descriptions advanced in the theory.

But Dickoff and James note that in practice disciplines such as nursing, as we have seen, more is needed than merely to describe the world. Any such theory 'must provide conceptualization specially intended to guide the shaping of reality to that profession's professional purpose' (ibid., p. 199). The theory must facilitate in some way the bringing about of the ends of the profession. As they say 'a good theory... is a theory that fulfils the purpose for which [it] was proposed or invented' (ibid., p. 198). This demands 'a conception of ends as well as means' (ibid., p. 199).

Dickoff and James claim a nursing theory should be 'situation producing' (1968, p. 198) (that is, it should show us how to produce the kinds of situations which match the ends of nursing). And, they write:

> Situation producing theories… attempt conceptualization of desired situations as
> well as conceptualizing the prescription under which an agent or practitioner must
> act in order to bring about situations of the kind conceived as desirable in the
> conception of the goal (1968, p. 200).

Put another way, such situation producing theories describe ('conceptualise') the ends of nursing, these being the relevant 'desired situations'. Also,
they describe ('conceptualise') the type of action ('prescription') which nurses
must perform in order to bring about those ends. So, put as crudely as
possible, a nursing theory must spell out the goals of nursing and the means
by which those goals are to be attained.

In addition to these two major components (the means-specification
component, and the ends-specification component) of a theory of nursing,
Dickoff and James posit a third component which they describe as a 'survey
list' (1968, p. 201). This

> calls attention to those aspects of activity and to those theories at whatever level
> deemed by the theorist relevant to the production of desired situations but not
> (or not yet) explicitly or fully incorporated into goal-content or prescriptions
> (ibid., p. 201).

This third component seeks to capture the kinds of phenomena which an
experienced nurse might invoke in her actions, aimed to meet the goals of
nursing, but not explicitly described in the prescriptive or means-stating
component of the theory. This might include, for example, prior knowledge
of the patient (see Dickoff and James's reference to 'internal resources of
agents' (1968, p. 201)). Hence at a general level the 'means' prescription
might require a nurse to give penicillin to a patient, but if the nurse is aware
that the patient is allergic to this, then she will not give it. At a different level,
a nurse's prior knowledge of an anxious patient may provide a source of information which she may recruit to calm down the patient.

This third 'catch all' component posited by Dickoff and James captures at
least partially what is discussed in Benner's idea of expertise. As we heard, for
Benner, the expert views situations in terms of mental patterns – gestalts –
which enable her to make expert judgements. And for Benner such capabili-
ties are not formulable, they are resistant to specification (perhaps even in principle for Benner). But Dickoff and James seem to leave open the possibility of
complete specification (1968, p. 201). They write: 'the basis of professional
judgement is incredibly complex and probably at no time fully articulate rather
than something mysterious, ineffable, or inborn' (ibid., p. 201). It seems
reasonable to conclude from this passage that they think the basis for such
judgements *can* be set out – that is, since they deny it is 'ineffable'.

So we have heard on Dickoff and James's account, a theory of nursing must have three components each of which specifies ends, means, and residual phenomena characteristic of professional judgement.

This specific conception of such a theory enables them to resist a familiar objection to the idea of a theory of nursing. According to the objection, since description is essentially the aim of theory, and since the aim of a nursing theory is not descriptive, it follows that there cannot be a theory of nursing. But as Dickoff and James illustrate, this objection presupposes an overly narrow conception of theory. According to their 'theory of theories' it is possible for theories to be more than merely descriptive. Theories can 'guide the shaping of reality to [a] profession's professional purpose' (1968, p. 199). Thus coherent sense is given to the idea of a theory with ends which are normative, rather than descriptive. Sense is given to the idea of a theory which seeks to bring about certain specified ends – to 'shape reality'.

This seems to me a perfectly acceptable conception of a nursing theory. It can be considered here as specifying conditions of adequacy which any such theory must meet.

It has just been seen how the conception of nursing theory developed by Dickoff and James can resist one objection stemming from the normative, as opposed to descriptive, ends of nursing. However, the evaluative nature of those ends does bring with it certain other difficulties. Recall that Dickoff and James's position on nursing theory refers to the need for a theory of nursing to shape reality to the ends of nursing. It is reasonable to conclude from this that, on their conception, there is some way of determining whether or not reality has in fact been so shaped, as they put it. A nurse may act as prescribed under the 'means' component of a nursing theory. The aim of the act is to shape reality in some way. As we have said, this amounts to trying to bring about the ends of nursing. So then we have to ask 'Has reality been shaped by nursing acts A, B, C, D, E and so on?' In other words has the patient's suffering been reduced? Has their quality of life been improved? Has their autonomy been fostered? Has their state of health been improved?

Our discussion in Chapters 5 and 7 strongly suggests that these questions cannot be answered independently of the views of the person concerned. Thus the question of whether the quality of life of a patient has been improved will require asking him. The reasons for this, as we heard, are twofold. First, improvement or deterioration in any phenomenological state (such as pain) can be discerned most authoritatively by the person in that state. There are no objective measures available to determine this. So with respect to the question of whether 'reality has been shaped' by a specific intervention there seems no objective way to confirm or falsify this in relation to phenomenological states.

Second, symptoms of illness are interpreted by patients in terms of their own self-projects. Thus, since once again they seem best placed to determine any improvements and deteriorations in their quality of life – that is, in terms of their specific narratives – there appear no objective measures available in order to determine whether or not interventions have 'shaped reality' in the desired way.

So a problem is this. One can never judge that 'reality has been shaped' by reference to an objectively available source of evidence. It will be necessary to be guided by the patient's own view. As noted previously, in a theory regarding the physical domain, or in applied science the question of whether 'reality has been shaped' can be determined in a way which is relatively unproblematic. The evidence relevant to the determination of the question is objectively available. But this is not so with reference to phenomenological states, and with reference to the perceived impact upon a 'self-project' of nursing interventions. Answers to these questions cannot be determined from the third-person perspective. Thus a theory requires generalisations, yet the need for narrative understanding and evaluation of phenomenological data entails that the applicability of a generalisation in any particular case cannot be known by 'objective' means.

Let us now try to make some progress beyond this apparent impasse. As mentioned above it is reasonable to take Dickoff and James's position to imply that a theory of nursing must require it to be possible to determine whether or not the ends of nursing have been obtained. Their view of a theory requires knowledge of whether or not 'reality has been shaped'. But due to the particular nature of nursing a problem arises in relation to the possibility of such knowledge. For it seems the question of whether or not the ends of nursing have been met is not open to objective determination. By 'objective' it is meant data which are accessible to all in the same way. But as seen, this is not so in nursing. The person who endures the pain is in a privileged position to determine whether or not his pain has subsided. And the same person appears in a privileged position to determine whether or not his self-project has been enhanced or jeopardised by nursing care.

The points we have made so far suggest that the question of whether or not 'reality has been shaped' is determined in individual cases by each patient. So does this, then, call into question the very idea of a theory of nursing? It does so only *if* the idea of objective verification is a necessary component of such a theory.

It was argued earlier that one cannot *know* how another is feeling, whether their suffering has been relieved and so on. Only they can know these things because only they have access to their mental states. Subjects also seem to have the same position of privileged access in relation to their narratives. They seem best placed to judge what matters most to them.

In response to this, it can be agreed that one cannot *know* what another is feeling in the way in which they themselves do. However, it is plain that certain factors would count as good evidence that a person is feeling anxious. They may say they are for example. Of course, they may be lying. Inevitably there is an epistemic gap between any judgement from the third-person perspective about the mental states of another person. But the existence of this gap need not preclude the making of judgements about the mental states of others, for example to the effect that they are in pain or are feeling anxious and so on. Such judgements can be plausible or otherwise, they may be wholly wrong, or they may be right, but they can be made. Given the presence of the epistemic gap, one cannot know with certainty what another is feeling, but one can make a judgement which is more or less plausible.

It is reasonable to suppose that in dealing with people in stressful situations that such situations present an opportunity for the development of the kinds of skills relevant to the making of judgements about the phenomenal states of others. The skilled nurse, through exposure and care about patients (and colleagues) in such situations, develops the kinds of patterns discussed by Benner. These enable such judgements to be made – they are not infallible, and are based upon discernible evidence, but they are in general reliable, hence the expert status of the nurse. (Although, recall our plea for modesty regarding the expert knowledge.)

Thus the fact of privileged access prevents our certain knowledge of the experiences of others, but need not prevent well-grounded judgements about them. These judgements are not infallible, but can be viewed in terms of grades of plausibility. Therefore this problem concerning the question of determining whether or not 'reality has been shaped' in accordance with the ends of nursing can be dealt with. In keeping with our conclusions regarding knowledge and persons, all the nurse has to go on here are interpretations. These will include a wide range of phenomena: what the patient says, what his physical signs are, how his body is presented (is the posture relaxed, or otherwise) and so on. But on the basis of these, a judgement can be made with regard to the success or otherwise of the nursing care delivered. Of course, the judgement may turn out to be mistaken. But this possibility need not prevent the making of judgements per se, and the possibility of evaluating between them in terms of their respective plausibility.

Consider now a further source of problems for the idea of a theory of nursing. The problem just discussed arose in relation to the ends of nursing – in relation to the determination of whether or not they have been met. Our next problem arises in relation to the means employed to bring about such ends. For surely such means must include generalisations over patients. Yet, this sits uncomfortably with what was said concerning the narrative conception of persons.

Generalisations and narratives

Generalisations at the biological level seem unlikely to have many exceptions: for example, humans have blood, humans bleed when blood vessels are pierced, humans need food, water and oxygen, and so on. So a place for such generalisations within a theory of nursing appears unproblematic.

Generalisations at a different level seem possible also, such as that represented in our 'principle of postural echo' (Chapter 3). Consider also generalisations such as humans grieve when they lose loved ones, humans prefer to be well rather than ill, humans seek comfort, humans seek human company, and so on *ad infinitum.*

Generalisations of these latter kind seem different from the former, biological generalisations in the sense that they are much more likely to have exceptions. A person may deliberately eschew human company, for example, in order to devote themselves to the worship of God; they may become a hermit. So a difference can be detected in terms of the confidence we can invest in these types of generalisations. Considerable confidence can be invested in the biological ones, less confidence in the latter kind.

What reason can be given for such an intuitively clear difference? One good reason is that the latter kinds of generalisations are more closely bound up with the narratives of persons. As the example of the hermit shows, his constituting an exception to the generalisation 'Humans seek the company of other humans' is due to the nature of his self-project. Any desire he has for the company of others is not considered by him to be as important as the desire to devote his life to the worship of God.

Our problem is that although the centrality of the notion of narrative generates problems with the inclusion of a role for generalisations within nursing, it is evident that generalisations are an essential component of a theory of nursing.

Suppose the theory includes a statement of the form 'if x do y'; for example, if a patient is anxious then speak to them (setting aside all the contextual details concerning whether the nurse has time that moment to speak to the patient and so on). For the sake of argument, let it be supposed that the aim is to reduce the level of the patient's anxiety. Here 'shaping reality' involves bringing about that state of affairs. Let us agree that objective measures such as a reduction in pulse rate are not sufficient to show that the patient's anxiety has decreased. Further, suppose that the anxiety reducing actions prescribed under x are generally thought to be successful. Of course the fact that acts of type x are generally successful does nothing to show that they will be successful in this particular case. There is a crucial difference between general and universal success.

Does the idea of a theory survive such contextual determination? In other words, suppose once more that in 80 per cent of cases acts of type x reduce anxiety. Knowing this will not guarantee that an act of type x will *in this instance* bring about a reduction in anxiety.

Yet surely the nurse who knows that acts of type x generally bring about reductions in anxiety levels is better prepared to help anxious patients than a nurse who knows no such general rules. So there seems some merit in learning and being able to put into practice general rules believed to foster the ends of nursing.

But can a collection of such generalisations, serving as the 'means' component of a theory of nursing, together with the other two components, constitute a theory of nursing? In a nursing theory the question of whether or not reality has been 'shaped' must be faced anew each time an act of a prescribed type is undertaken. This is an unavoidable feature of the contextualised nature of nursing. But our last deliberations seem to suggest that generalisations can be useful, can help bring about the ends of nursing. So can we now decide whether this contextual feature of nursing (that is, that it cannot be known in advance whether a successful generalisation will be successful in a particular case) jeopardises the very idea of a nursing theory?

Recall what was said earlier concerning a theory of asthma. This would require:

1. a description of the condition
2. a specification of its causes, and
3. a specification of the mechanisms by which these causes lead to the development of the condition.

Points 1 to 3 would generate explanations and predictions.

Applied to the idea of a nursing theory, (1) is equivalent to the specification of ends. (2) is equivalent to the specification of causes in that it specifies the conditions implicated in the bringing about of (1). And (3) can be understood as the conditions which explicate the relations between (1) and (2).

Thus, take Benner and Wrubel's theory as an example of a nursing theory. The relevant ends (1) can be as in our earlier example, relieving the anxiety of a patient. The means (2) involve a general rule to the effect that anxiety often relates to patients' interpretations of their symptoms. The explicating relationship between (1) and (2) is achieved by (3). And this can be understood in terms of our narrative conception of the person, in which, as we heard, persons are constituted by a narrative. Thus symptoms are interpreted in terms of their perceived impact upon the patient's self-project (both by the patient and by his relatives). It should be stressed of course that the generalisations which figure in a nursing theory will be more complex and numerous than those given here.

With regard to what can be generalised from one patient to another, by a nurse, Gadow suggests that any knowledge gained by the nurse in the course of engagement with a patient is not generalisable. She says it is 'general without being generalisable' (1995, p. 43). The sense in which such knowledge is general for Gadow is that it stems from the contributions of both parties (nurse and patient), and is greater than the sum of what each brings to the interactions. Thus she writes 'The meaning expressed in the [co-authored] narrative is general in that it transcends the singularity of each author – nurse and client – at the same time that it remains particular to their situation' (1995, p. 42).

So such knowledge is general, as noted, in that it is greater than the contributions of each individual. But surely, one wants to say against Gadow, there is a clear sense in which the knowledge obtained by the nurse is (at least) *relevant* to subsequent patients that she might come across. Thus recall the point that was made earlier in discussion of Benner's claims about expert nurses. While it can be allowed that no two cases are the same, the expert nurse hones her 'pattern recognition' skills in her dealings with patients. It seems plausible to suppose the nurse transfers something across from caring for earlier patients and those she meets later in her career. This is not to say that the later cases are replicas of the earlier cases and so the nurse simply generalises to later cases strategies found successful in earlier ones. Rather, the way the nurse deals with later cases is informed, however subtly, by her dealings with earlier cases. This capacity for such fine-tuned judgement, I take it, is one of the components of expert practice.

Thus one is not 'beginning anew' so to speak with each patient one meets. If the patients are relevantly similar, in some respects, it is reasonable to judge that the way the nurse cares for a later patient can be affected by her nursing of an earlier patient. Of course the nurse might act differently, or act in the same way given her judgement that there is some relationship of similarity between the present patient and the past one.

We began this discussion of the relations between particular cases and generalisations with a fairly rough and ready distinction between generalisations at the biological level, and those more closely bound to the narratives of people.

It was suggested earlier that generalisations at the biological level are much less likely to have exceptions than those at the narratival level. Thus the claim 'humans seek oxygen' seems exceptionless, but the claim 'humans grieve when they lose loved ones' although generally true, may have exceptions (for example psychopaths might be exceptions to this). It should not be concluded from this distinction that the two realms are in fact wholly separable; and it will be pertinent to make some further points on the relations between them here.

Recall the point that generalisations need to be interpreted in the context of a particular patient's narrative. If we do this, even the apparently unassailable generalisation 'humans seek oxygen' can be shown to be problematic. For there may be cases in which a person expressly refuses oxygen. For example, suppose a person has a chronic, severe breathing problem now in its terminal phase. The person requests that no oxygen be given to them. They simply want to be left to die.

Similar problems arise for generalisations such as 'humans seek food'. Hunger strikers and people with *anorexia nervosa* generate exceptions to this.

These examples show how the narrative level impinges on the biological. For in health care work, as argued in Chapter 5 above, the biological understanding we have is not obtained for its own sake but for health-related ends. And it is reasonable to characterise such ends in narrative terms – that is, in terms of the capacity of a person to pursue activities they wish to.

In response to this problem regarding generalisations at the biological level, it may be suggested that at a lower level, so to speak, at the level of physiological processes – body chemistry and physics – generalisations *are* in fact exceptionless.

However, even here there are problems with such a claim. Even here, it can be argued, the level of narrative understanding impinges. Thus for example it is common to say that a patient's attitude to their illness is not irrelevant to its course. Thus a person who has 'given up', it is said, is likely to die more quickly than a person, in a roughly similar predicament, but who has a strong desire to live. Reportedly, the attitude of a sufferer to an illness may affect the rate at which, say, a wound heals. (See, for example, Revans, 1964; Wulff, 1994.)

If such data are reliable, it suggests that even this deepest of biological levels is not immune from narrative-bound considerations. For reports appear to suggest that a sense of hopelessness on the part of a person has an effect on what seem to be purely biological phenomena, immune from the realm of narratival understanding. But this is not so, apparently.

It is not clear to me whether this kind of phenomena exemplifies mind–body causation, or supports the Merleau-Pontian position in which persons are 'body-subjects'. Either way, it strongly supports the position that narratival understanding is of great significance to nursing, and to health care work in general.

In further support of that claim, recall points we made earlier in discussion of Benner and Wrubel's theory. It was pointed out there that significant numbers of health problems (perhaps all) are related to the narratives of their sufferers. Thus diseases relating to lifestyles involving smoking, unhealthy diet, heavy drinking and so on, seem plainly bound to the narratives of their sufferers, to their self-projects and the self-conceptions which fuel these.

If these points concerning the pervasive character of narrative-bound considerations are accepted, clearly the importance of further work on the nature of narrative is required. But further, problems regarding generalisations seem accentuated. For as we have seen, any generalisation at the biolog ical level – even at the 'deepest' part of this level – may not be immune from narrative-bound considerations. Nonetheless, as shown here, the place of generalisations within nursing can be defended. Even though on a particular occasion the nurse does not know whether application of the generalisation will be successful, it seems reasonable to judge that a nurse who has knowledge of relevant generalisations is better placed to nurse appropriately than one who lacks them.

Two further problems

We now consider two further obstacles to the idea of a nursing theory. The first is in relation to means. This problem arises since it may be thought that a theory of how to bring about certain situations requires a specification of the steps needed to actually bring those situations about. But the view that practical knowing resists specification, and the view that nursing knowledge is 'invisible' (Liaschenko, 1998) seem to show such specification is not possible. Thus can a theory of nursing survive these challenges?

The second problem stems from the wide diversity of nursing. Does this not entail there cannot be a theory of nursing?

(i) Can the 'means' be specified?

Recall that in Dickoff and James's view, a nursing theory can be specified in principle. Yet, in Chapter 3, we allowed that a relatively robust distinction can be made between propositional and practical knowing such that knowing how is not reducible to knowing that. There will always be elements of practical knowing which remain elusive to the task of specification of them. Moreover, recall, Ryle argues persuasively that propositional knowing, in fact, presupposes practical knowing.

Further, Liaschenko (1998) argues that much of what she calls nursing knowledge is 'invisible'. By this it is meant that since it is not recognisably medical knowledge, it is not regarded as knowledge. For example, she discusses 'knowledge of how to get things done' (ibid., pp. 14–16). Among other things, this involves 'connecting the patient to resources' (ibid., p. 15). One of the skills of a good, experienced nurse is to have a good knowledge of matters which might seem peripheral to the task of nursing patients. Such knowledge includes: awareness of which doctors respond quickly when asked to do so, and which don't; which porters one can rely on to know the location of scarce equipment; which contacts among colleagues to exploit in order to obtain materials one is short of (for example sterile dressings, bed linen), and so on. In short, Liaschenko draws attention to a range of knowledge which an experienced nurse will accumulate and draw upon in her practice. This range will extend far beyond the parameters of the ward upon which she works, if she is ward based, or her immediate colleagues, in other nursing contexts.

Can the coherence of the idea of a theory of nursing survive these two points: first that deriving from the irreducibility of practical knowing to propositional knowing; and second that deriving from the 'invisibility' of nursing knowledge?

It seems plain that accepting the irreducibility of practical knowing to propositional knowing is incompatible with Dickoff and James's view of nursing theory. For as we saw above, this is such that all components of the theory are specifiable. However, need this threaten the whole idea of a theory of nursing?

My suggestion is that it need not, given a suitably qualified sense of the term 'theory'. We noted the three components of theory above:

1. the conditions aimed at;

2. the 'conditions' which bring about the conditions aimed at; and

3. the mechanism or better, the rationalising considerations which make intelligible the relations between (1) and (2). This was exemplified briefly above with reference to Benner and Wrubel's theory of nursing.

The qualifications needed are these. First, it is evident that wholesale specification of the conditions referred to in (2) will not be possible. In other words, there cannot be a 'step-by-step' instruction manual knowledge of which will be sufficient to enable one to be a good nurse. Given the distinction between practical and propositional knowledge, the possession of mere propositional knowledge will not be sufficient to bring about the ends of nursing. Knowledge of how to effect relevant propositional knowledge will be required and this, it is reasonable to suppose, can be acquired only by practice. So a theory of nursing will not be a complete instruction manual. (To take a related example, propositional knowledge of the steps involved in wheelbuilding is soon shown to fall short of knowledge of how to build a wheel once one tries.)

Also, recall what was said earlier concerning individual responses to illness, and the importance of the self-projects of patients. As brought out in several places in our discussions herein, two patients may have the same physical complaint yet it does not follow that they should be nursed in the same way. Moreover, even if it is accepted that a place for generalisations is appropriate, due to the last point, on any particular occasion the generalisation a nurse takes to be relevant, may turn out not to be. Thus recall our hypothetical 'principle of postural echo' referred to earlier (Chapter 3). As a generalisation this may be stated thus: 'anxious people tend to adopt the posture of the person with whom they are interacting'.

Of course this need not be cast in universal form, such that it is being claimed as true for *all* anxious people. Rather, it is claimed as a generalisation true of many cases, for the sake of argument, let us say *most* (that is, in other words, it applies in more than half of cases).

Suppose, then, a nurse comes to learn this and applies it, as described in our earlier discussion. Of course one can accept the plausibility of the generalisation *and* accept that its general plausibility does not entail its success in every case, just in many cases. So, as noted earlier, on any particular occasion the generalisation may not apply successfully, may not be confirmed.

But as we saw, this in turn, does not thereby entail that the generalisation is of no use whatsoever to the nurse. It seems perfectly reasonable to suppose that a nurse who is aware of, and can apply, the generalisation is better equipped to help a person cope with anxiety than a nurse who is unaware of the generalisation. (Assuming, for the sake of argument here that the application of the principle does allay anxiety, that this is a plausibly good thing to aim at, and that some rationalising factor can explicate the link between relaxed posture and lowering of anxiety.)

So what is being claimed here then is that acceptance of the individual nature of responses to illness need not be taken to generate a fatal blow to the attempt to devise a theory of nursing. Nor need the fact that a theory can contain only generalisations, not universalisations (that is, statements true in all cases). And lastly, the fact that a theory cannot exhaustively specify all components of nursing actions again need not be taken to threaten the whole idea of a theory of nursing. It should, however, be recognised that the implementation of the theory requires more than the learning of the propositions which compose it. This stems from the point that practical and propositional knowledge differ importantly.

So the points which may be taken to call into question the idea of a theory of nursing so far discussed include: the ineffability of (at least some) practical knowledge; and the fact of individualised responses to illness. Concessions have been made such that the ineffability of practical knowledge is compatible with the idea of a theory. The presence of generalisations within a theory is compatible with the fact of individualised responses to illness. On any particular case, generalisations may fail to apply, but as shown in the 'postural echo' example this need not entail the uselessness of such generalisations, for example in terms of their general employment in bringing about desired ends.

It is worth adding a comment here regarding the relationship between such generalisations and the features of expert practice which we noted in discussion of Benner's work (Chapter 3).

As a novice, generalisations such as the principle just discussed may be learned. They are put into practice, initially consciously, but as experience develops they become part of the therapeutic repertoire of the nurse, and can be enacted unreflectively. Of course, strictly speaking, each situation which the nurse encounters is a unique event. By definition, it is an event which has not happened previously (unless the nurse is a time traveller!). Hence some judgement is required on the part of the nurse that a later situation is relevantly similar to an earlier one such that the generalisation is enacted, albeit unreflectively, on the part of the nurse.

In Benner's terms, the situation is perceived in terms of relevant 'patterns' by the expert. It is these which unreflectively bring about the nurse's employment of the relevant aspect of his therapeutic repertoire. As Benner notes, the generalisations are constantly modified and honed in the light of experience of their application. Again this is not necessarily done consciously. Aspects of generalisations are transferred from previously experienced cases to later cases. Thus the generalisations acquire a subtlety of discernment as the nurse's experience grows. They are initially coarse, and gradually refined.

Before moving on, we noted earlier Liaschenko's point concerning the invisibility of much nursing knowledge. Part of this is practical knowing and hence non-specifiable. So it cannot feature in a theory of nursing. But other parts of it would seem to be specifiable, for example relating to typical features of institutions, and relating to communication skills. There seems no reason why these 'invisible' items of nursing knowledge cannot be placed within Dickoff and James's 'survey list'.

Lastly, what of the moral component of nursing? Given acceptance of the idea that generalisations have a place within nursing, similar points relating to the 'postural echo' principle can be made here. It can be useful for nurses to learn to apply even generalisations about moral matters, for example 'respect the wishes of patients'. As before, this is not a universal claim, only a general one. It can be applied in the same way as the 'postural echo' generalisation. For example, if a patient wishes to be given information which a nurse thinks will be harmful to the patient, her initial reaction may be to withhold it. But if the nurse is persuaded of the legitimacy of the generalisation just given, she may suppress her own intuition and act in accord with the learned generalisation. As before, this will gradually be inculcated into the nurse's therapeutic repertoire so there will be no need to rehearse the generalisation in all cases where the question of its applicability arises. It will be manifested in the nurse's store of practical knowledge. Thus of course, the moral aspect of nursing will not all be specifiable, the kinds of emotional response discussed by Nortvedt (1996, 1998) and Scott (2000) (Chapter 6 above) seem crucial elements of morality, and seem likely to resist specification. But as with the discussion of the postural echo principle, this need not be taken to subvert the very idea of a theory of nursing: not all aspects of nursing will be specified in the theory. It will contain a general conception of ends, means, and the rationalising factors which relate means and ends.

(ii) The diversity of nursing

A further challenge to the very idea of a theory of nursing has been developed by Cash (1990). Drawing upon the work of Wittgenstein, Cash argues persuasively that nursing is a 'family resemblance' concept. Thus there is no single feature common to all areas of nursing. Rather, there are a series of overlapping aspects, as Wittgenstein puts it: 'a complicated network of similarities overlapping and criss-crossing' (1953, para. 66). So, for example, Orem's characterisation of nursing in terms of 'the substitution of self-care agency in the presence of a self-care deficit' (Cash, 1990, p. 252) should not be seen to be unique to nursing. For, as he says, medical personnel are also involved in such a role.

Further, think of the range of activities and contexts of nursing practice: the ICU, a community home with people with mild learning disabilities, and so on. Is it feasible to suppose there will be one theory applicable to all these diverse areas?

In response to this challenge, note that Cash's position only rules out a general theory of nursing. So the acceptance of Cash's case need not rule out a less general theory, for example one related to ICU nursing or mental health nursing. But further, Cash's position only rules out a general theory of nursing if one ties this to the idea that there is a specific range of activities unique to nursing, and found in all areas of nursing. So a general theory which did not take on the claim that it applied only to nursing would still be possible.

Thus consider again Benner and Wrubel's theory. The ends are helping people cope with the stress of illness. The means include grasping the self-conceptions of patients. The rationalising element stems from the narrative view of the person. There is no compelling reason why one could not, *in principle*, accept this as both a theory of nursing and a theory of medicine; in other words, it could stand as a general theory of health care work. This is compatible with its being a theory of nursing.

However, in practice, there do seem difficulties in regarding Benner and Wrubel's theory as applicable in all areas of nursing. For example in work with people with intellectual disabilities, it is far from clear that such people count as ill, or that they have any health-related problem (Nordenfelt, 1993). On the agreement they are not ill, it follows that Benner and Wrubel's theory cannot apply since the ends at which it aims are not appropriate to working with people with intellectual disabilities. For it seems that Benner and Wrubel's starting point is that people with whom the nurse comes into contact in the course of her work have a health problem. It is a matter of considerable debate as to whether intellectual disability amounts to a health problem. To show why, if briefly, recall that on the narrative conception of the person, the significance of illness stems from its perceived impact upon that narrative: will one be able to pursue the goals important to one? But clearly a person can have an intellectual disability and this need not have any adverse affect on their capacity to pursue the goals they value. Hence Benner and Wrubel's theory does not seem to apply here.

This shows only that Benner and Wrubel's theory does not count as a general theory of nursing. It does not show that there cannot be such a theory – although, as noted, Cash's case strongly suggests that any such theory should resist the temptation to claim it rests upon a foundation unique to nursing; or that the theory itself applies uniquely to nursing.

So the idea of a theory of nursing, it appears, can be defended from these last two challenges, and the others described in this chapter. It should be stressed that here we are not trying to set out a theory of nursing. Our purpose is to show that certain apparent obstacles to the development of such a theory can be overcome. Thus, it seems, the 'unity requirement' character-istic of practices can be met.

In summary, then, of this attempt to preserve the idea of nursing as a prac-tice by defending the coherence of the idea of a theory of nursing: we noted that a theory requires three components relating to ends, means and a way of rationalising the relations between these. We drew attention to a non-arbitrary, if fallible way in which it can be determined whether or not the ends of nursing have been met – that is, by recruiting evidence, although admittedly 'evidence' in a much weaker sense than the sense of this in the natural sciences. We distinguished generalisations from universalisations and allowed a place for the former within nursing. And the idea of the person as a narrative was said to provide the rationalising link between these prior two components. Prior chapters have raised the difficulty of applying such a conception of the person to cases such as nursing those in PVS. In response, it was suggested the idea of a plight can be extended to such patients to explain why there is a moral pull to care for such patients, although, it has to be conceded, problems remain in applying the idea of a theory of nursing to these patients, for example regarding ends and so on. When have the ends of nursing been met in the nursing care of such patients?

Before moving off the topic of nursing theory it is worth making one last observation. This concerns the marked contrast between the nursing and medical literature on the topic of theory. While nursing literature is replete with theories of nursing and discussions of these, no similar literature exists within medicine. Why is there this marked discrepancy? I do not have a ready explanation. One possibility is that the medical enterprise is so closely aligned with natural science that it has been taken for granted that any attempt to devise a theory of medicine need only invoke components of a relevant natural science, for example biology. However, as mentioned, I will not pursue this question further, save to note this striking difference between nursing and medical literatures (see also Wulff et al., 1986).

SUGGESTIONS FOR FURTHER READING

It is difficult to know where to begin to refer readers to books on nursing theory. I find McKenna (1997) helpful and clear. King and Fawcett (1997) is a useful collection; as indeed is Parse (1987).

Philosophical discussion on the idea of theory, like Hempel's (1996) classic, tends to be difficult. See also, Chapters 8 and 9 of Chalmers (1999); and of course, Dickoff and James (1968) as discussed in the text.

Conclusion

Following a general introductory chapter we discussed the concept of know-ledge. In the realms of both practical and propositional knowledge a concep-tion of knowledge was supported such that it should be conceived of as essentially revisable. Thus, it was argued, an attitude of modesty towards what we think we know is the proper attitude to be adopted by practitioners and theorists alike. We should be sensitive to the possibility that what we currently regard as knowledge may be shown to be false at some later time. And also sensitive to the possibility that novel views are conceived of in terms of currently favoured ones. This may entail that novel views are not given a fair hearing, they may simply be evaluated in ways which presuppose acceptance of our currently held views. A fine balance is required here to ensure a will-ingness to consider novel views and at the same time to respect the virtue of 'conservatism' put forward by Quine and Ullian, and endorsed here.

Within the domain of practical knowledge it proved possible to articulate a distinction analogous to that within the realm of propositional knowledge relating to degrees of plausibility. Benner's five stages in the route from novice to expert were invoked to set this out. This helped to explain why the perfor-mance of the expert is more likely to be successful than that of the novice. Even within this realm, it should be remembered, an attitude of modesty is appropriate in relation to one's expertise. As we saw, what counts as expert practice is itself bound to current standards and conceptions of means and ends. Since these are not immutable, modesty is motivated.

Our discussion then centred on the idea of a person in nursing. Consider-ation of four main responses to the mind–body problem left us with two possible candidates. Although neither is without problems, we favoured a 'dependence view' over a Merleau-Pontian view on grounds of conservatism. The dependence view, it was claimed, has the merits which have led theorists to reject Cartesian and crude reductionist views of mind and body, without requiring the wholesale conceptual revision entailed by acceptance of the Merleau-Pontian position. Given acceptance of an ontology of the person such that persons are beings with both mental and physical properties, the subject of the identities of particular persons was turned to, and a narrative concep-tion of this put forward. In this, the identity of persons is described by a narra-tive which is a description of the pursuance of a self-project. This view of the person was shown to have especial relevance to nursing. In nursing, narrative understanding of patients seems crucial to the proper care of them. There proved to be problems with such a position relating to care of PVS patients. Such patients appear to fall outside of the ontology of persons. In partial

192

response it was suggested that the ontological place of PVS patients, in itself, entails no moral directives concerning how they ought to be regarded. And also, such patients have a 'plight' in an attenuated sense at least, and have a narrative history, although it must be added, there is nothing that it is *like* to be in PVS (if the medical definition of this condition is correct).

Our discussion of care attempted to clarify the usual 'intentional' sense of care, but also to clarify a less understood 'ontological' sense of care. As seen, care is a feature of all humans in this ontological sense. Moreover, articulation of care in the 'identity-constituting' sense, helped to make sense of Benner and Wrubel's claims regarding the centrality – *primacy* – of caring to nursing. Although, it should be added, neither intentional nor ontological care could be shown unique to nursing, they do seem necessary components of it. In nursing, it is necessary to undertake acts of intentional caring, and to focus these in a way bound to the identity-constituting sense of care. This discussion helps bring out the moral dimension of nursing also. Acts of intentional care owe their intelligibility to a recognition of the vulnerability of humans to pain and suffering.

Equipped with an account of knowledge, an ontology of the person, and having made some progress in articulation of the idea of care we turned to discuss the nature of nursing. Conditions of adequacy for any such account emerge from our discussion hitherto: any such account must allow a view of knowledge such that it is revisable, and such that practical knowledge has a central place. Any account of nursing must respect the views advanced here concerning the nature of the person. And the same applies in relation to the notion of care. Thus our view concerning knowledge, our view concerning the centrality of interpretation, and the moral component of nursing as revealed in our discussion of intentional care must all be respected by any account of nursing. It is with such considerations in mind that we considered 'class inclusion' claims such that nursing is a science, an art or a practice.

It transpired that the attempt to identify nursing with science is deeply problematic. This is in part due to the role of knowledge in each, in science it is primarily of intrinsic value, but in nursing it is of instrumental value. Even the conception of nursing as an applied science proved implausible due to the nature of the objects of applied science. These it seems, are essentially such that items of a kind all exhibit the same properties. Thus, as argued, there is no requirement to treat individual pieces of copper, say, differently – as *individuals*. Yet this is key to nursing, as the narrative account of the person shows. Further differences centre on the moral dimension of nursing, its interpretive complexity and the inescapable place of subjective data. We were able to deal more quickly and to reject the view of nursing as an art. Such a view may recapture some of the important aspects of nursing masked by the conception of nursing as a science, for example the realm of practical knowing, but as we saw, art focuses on the emotions of the artist in a way which is incompatible with nursing. Art seems essentially self-regarding while nursing is essentially other-regarding. Morcover, a moral dimension is at most a contingent feature of art, but is a necessary feature of nursing.

The final option considered here is that nursing is a practice in the sense articulated by MacIntyre. It proved possible to make this case without doing violence to either concept, although, as we saw it proved necessary to shore up the 'unity' requirement on practices in our final chapter. Key elements of nursing, relating to our enquiries within epistemology, ontology and value-enquiry proved possible to encompass within the conception of nursing as a practice. For example, an explicit moral component is claimed for a practice. And the idea that practices are in continuous development – are extended arguments – sits well with the view of knowledge favoured within this book. The idea of a practice also seems rich enough to encompass the practical aspect of nursing, in the technical and interpretive senses of this, and also in the practical realm considered more broadly (for example in connection with activities such as managing a caseload and so on).

We saw in our final chapter that the unifying of means and ends charac-teristic of practices, and nursing theory, can survive some of the implications of points made hitherto regarding the narrative conception of the person.

Finally, it follows from what has been said about practices that the present work, at most, can be expected to provide only a contribution to the further development of nursing as a practice. There are many issues which there has not been time to raise, and many that have been raised need further discus-sion. However, there is only a limited amount that a single text can aim to do. And it is hoped that this present work will provoke others to improve upon it and contribute further to the topic of philosophy of nursing.

Glossary

It should be stressed that probably all the entries given in the glossary can be challenged. Given this, readers may find other reference sources such as Flew (1979) or Honderich (1992) worth consideration. Of course the same proviso occurs in relation to these sources also.

Aesthetics The enquiry into values such as beauty, and more generally into the properties we ascribe to works of art such as paintings, poems, novels, and so on.

Care Ontological care is divided into two kinds: deep and identity-constituting (see Chapter 7). 'Deep' care refers to the fact of the world's inescapably mattering to us (for example at the biological level). Identity-constituting care concerns the sense in which we are 'constituted by our cares'. Intentional care concerns particular caring acts undertaken in response to the vulnerability of others.

Contingent truth In contrast to necessary truths, which describe that which *could not* be otherwise, contingent truths describe that which *could be* otherwise. Thus it is a contingent truth about the number 4 that I always select it when doing the national lottery. I happen to choose that number, but clearly I may have chosen some other number, or not do the lottery at all.

Epistemology That part of philosophy concerned with the concept of knowledge: what it is, whether it is possible to obtain it, whether there are special sources of it (such as intuition or introspection), and so on. (See Chapters 2 and 3.)

Ethics The enquiry into values such as moral rightness and wrongness.

Intentional states Mental states such as beliefs, desires and fears. Intentional acts derive from intentional states.

Interpretivism Minimally, the view that all accounts of reality, descriptions of experience, theories and so on are interpretations.

Knowledge Propositional knowledge has a necessary relationship to truth such that if a claim is known, necessarily, it is true. (This is not the case with belief.) Practical knowledge concerns 'know-how', for example as is manifested in the performance of practical skills and tasks.

Logic The enquiry into the nature of argumentation.

Narrative The life story of a person. It should be stressed there is little likelihood of there being 'one true' narrative; much more likely – probably inevitably – is the presence of different, competing stories.

Narrative understanding Understanding persons in terms of their life story, of what is important to them (in contrast to biological understanding).

Necessary and sufficient conditions *x* is a *necessary* condition of A if A cannot occur in the absence of *x*. *x* is a *sufficient* condition of A if the presence of *x* guarantees the presence of A. Thus oxygen is a necessary condition for the presence of fire (apparently, fire requires the presence of oxygen); but clearly oxygen is not a sufficient condition for the presence of fire!

Necessary truth A statement which describes a necessary feature of a thing; a characteristic which it cannot help but instance, which could not be otherwise. For example '2 is an even number' is a necessary truth. In this book it has been claimed that the statement 'Nursing is a moral response to human vulnerability' is a necessary truth.

Ontology That part of philosophy concerned with existence questions. For example, what distinguishes things which do exist from those which do not? What is it to be one thing as opposed to another? What is the relationship between classes of things, for example persons, and their members? (See Chapters 4 and 5.)

Phenomenology A philosophical programme which aims to describe human experience as it really is, undistorted by the lens of scientific, philosophical, or common-sense categories. (See esp. Merleau-Ponty, 1962, p. vii; and E. Husserl 'Phenomenology' in *Encyclopaedia Britannica*, 14th edn, pp. 699–702.)

Phenomenology When it is said of mental states that they have a phenomenology, it is meant that there is a way it 'feels' to have them, and which (at least) partly defines them – such states include pain, and fear.

Philosophy of nursing The examination of philosophical problems as these bear upon or are raised by nursing theory and practice. (See Chapter 1.)

Plight The morally salient features of a human being's predicament.

Positivism A programme within philosophy of science the intention of which is to place scientific findings on a secure footing, to give them a 'positive basis'. (See Chapter 8.)

Realism Ontological realism is the view that the world exists independently of the existence of human beings. In realist approaches to science it is characteristically held that the business of the scientist is to describe this independently-existing world. (See Chapter 8.)

Reductionism The attempt to show that one kind of thing or property, 'really is' nothing more than another apparently distinct kind of thing or property. For example that the mind is nothing but the brain; or that mental properties are nothing but physical ones, and so on.

Self-conception A person's view of the kind of person they are, or aspire to be – a view which 'fuels' a self-project.

Self-project That which is described in the narrative of a person.

Supervenience A relationship between types of properties, specifically a relationship of dependence. (See Chapter 4.)

Notes

Chapter 1

1. One of Quine's (1951) suggestions is that our beliefs can be envisaged through the metaphor of a web. At the centre of this web are beliefs which we would be very reluctant to give up. They are beliefs the truth of which we are especially certain. Thus for example, '2 + 2 = 4' might be one such belief, as might the belief that other people exist, or that objects fall when they are dropped, or that London is the capital of the UK, or that humans need oxygen, and so on. At the periphery of the web we have beliefs about which we are less confident, for example that tomorrow it will rain, or that one is a good judge of character, or that one's football team will win the FA Cup, and so on. As Quine puts it, beliefs which lie at the centre of the web are the ones which possess greatest immunity to revision. They are the beliefs the truth of which we have most confidence in and only remarkable circumstances would persuade us to revise them, and judge them to be false.

   We can think of concepts in this way too. Thus suppose we think of each specific concept as a web. Certain things will be central to that concept and others peripheral. The central elements will be the defining features of it.

   We can understand philosophical enquiry as attempting to identify those things which are central to a concept. Doing this enables us to distinguish elements which are central from elements which are peripheral. Hence we can think of philosophical enquiry as trying to uncover that which is true of anything which falls under a concept, by definition, as it were. Thus it can be said that anyone who understands the concept also knows that much about any instance of it. For example, the claim that nursing involves the performance of caring actions seems a credible candidate for a necessary truth about nursing. So if anyone knew the meaning of the word 'nursing' they would understand that nursing involves the performance of caring actions.

   This centre/periphery distinction may also be expressed by the distinction between that which is necessarily true of the things which fall under a concept and that which is contingently true of the things which fall under a concept.

   Thus, on the supposition that the performance of caring actions is a necessary feature of nursing, it follows that in order to nurse one is required to perform such acts. This we can cast as a necessary truth: unavoidably, if N is a nurse, N is expected to perform caring acts. But having red hair seems plainly to be a contingent truth about any nurse; one can be a nurse with any colour hair, but one cannot be a nurse and not be expected to perform caring acts.

   We are here articulating a distinction between (a) that which lies at the centre of a concept, and thus contributes to its nature, partially defines it. And (b) that which is at the *periphery* of a concept, and thus not definitive of it.

197

As will be seen later in our discussion of care, and of the nature of nursing, the distinction is of crucial significance. For claims that caring defines nursing, or that nursing is a science, or is an art, are claims about what lies at the very centre of the concept of nursing. To substantiate such claims it has to be shown that they are in fact defining, and not peripheral, are necessary, not contingent truths about nursing. Yet as we will see evidence in support of these claims often supports only the claim that art or science, or caring is contingently related to nursing, and not necessarily. For example (and to anticipate our later discussion), the fact that nurses use art therapeutically may be a contingent truth about nursing. This does not entail the necessary truth that, by definition, nursing is an art.

Chapter 2

1. It should be said that this last passage raises some deep and difficult problems. The philosophical position being criticised in the text is that of subjectivism. See Edwards, 1990 for a thorough survey of types of subjectivism and relativism.

Chapter 3

1. Regarding the more general sense of practical knowledge, see Aristotle on *phronesis*, as explained by, Dunne, 1993; also see Heidegger, 1962 and his claims on 'circumspection'.

Chapter 4

1. For ease of exposition I have deliberately omitted to discuss the distinction between the self and the person. This would generate too much complexity for a text such as this, although it signals an area in need of further work (see, for example, Merrill, 1998).

2. By 'disease' I mean to refer to the physical lesions or abnormalities which are commonly taken to cause, or at least underlie, feelings of ill health. Thus a broken bone, a virus, and failure of kidney function all count as diseases as these are construed here. By 'illness' it is meant the kind of feeling of ill health which typically leads us to suppose we are not well or need some medical assistance. So illness and disease are clearly separable in that one may have a disease, for example a virus, but not feel ill. And one may feel ill without there being an underlying disease.

3. More technically, it appears that intentional states are essentially relational in the sense that their identities depend upon things outside the brain, but brain states themselves are not essentially relational, their identities do not depend upon the environment of their bearer (that is, the thinker).

Chapter 6

1. The expression 'intentional care' is being used here to refer to caring acts which are deliberately, consciously undertaken by people. This kind of care will be contrasted

later with ontological caring. An example of the kind of act I have in mind here is an act such as, say, helping a frail person who has just fallen over to stand up again. Here one makes a decision to act in that way and does so. It should be said that this picture of acts of intentional care is not straightforward. For it has seemed to some, plausibly, that caring acts can stem from a kind of 'reflex' action, one which *need not* issue from a conscious decision. Nonetheless I take it that the description of caring acts of the former kind – those one decides to undertake – will be sufficiently familiar to readers. And so such acts will be our focus here. Ultimately, I would argue that caring acts of the 'reflex' kind stem from an initial phase of acting in which the actor consciously decides to undertake a caring act. Such acts then become habitual in some people, much as virtues are claimed by some to be habits in a closely related sense.

Chapter 8

1. Our term 'science' derives from the Latin *scientia* which in turn derives from the ancient Greek *episteme*. It is this last term which is rendered as science in translations of Aristotle's work. And it is this conception of science which is appealed to in order to sustain the broad view. Aristotle held there to be three 'bodies of knowledge', practical, productive and theoretical. These cover the fields of ethics and politics (practical), cobbling, farming, tailoring and medicine (productive), and mathematics, natural science, theology and philosophy (theoretical). Hence my characterisation of it here as supporting a broad conception of science. See Aristotle's *Metaphysics*, Bk. VI, 1025b 25 (Ackrill, 1987, p. 279) for the threefold division of knowledge. See also Ackrill's glossary in which the term 'episteme' can be translated variously as 'knowledge, scientific knowledge, branch of knowledge, science, understanding' (p. xiv).

2. It is also claimed that science, in addition to description, aims at explanation and prediction. But these seem logically secondary to, parasitic upon, description. Explanation presupposes accurate description, as does prediction. (Unless one favours an instrumentalist account of science.)

3. Other tenets include commitment to hypothetico-deductive model of explanation in science. This is a model of explanation in which explanations take the form of arguments (in the philosophical sense) with premises and a conclusion. For example, suppose the event to be explained (or predicted) is an unconscious, frail, patient developing a pressure sore. The explanation of this may have the following form:

    (a) An unconscious frail patient, Smith, has been lying in the same position for several days.
    (b) Blood supply to pressure areas has been cut off.
    (c) Tissue necroses in the absence of blood supply. Therefore
    (d) Smith has developed a pressure sore.

    If (a), (b) and (c) are true, (d) necessarily follows. This model can be 'backward looking' that is, to explain events which have already occurred. Or it can be 'forward-looking' and predict future events – unless we give Smith pressure area care, he'll develop a pressure sore. See Hempel, 1966.

Bibliography

Ackrill J.L. (ed.) (1987) *A New Aristotle Reader* (Oxford: Clarendon Press).

Aggleton P. and Chalmers H. (1986) *Nursing Models and the Nursing Process* (London: Macmillan – now Palgrave).

Alston W.P. (1971) 'Varieties of privileged access', *American Philosophical Quarterly*, 8: 223–41.

Aristotle *Ethics* (trans.) J.A.K. Thomson (1953) (Harmondsworth: Penguin).

Aristotle, *Poetics* (abridged version in Ackrill (1987), pp. 540–56).

Armstrong D.M. (1968) *A Materialist Theory of Mind* (London: RKP).

Asimov I. (1984) *Asimov's Guide to Science* (Harmondsworth: Penguin).

Audi R. (1998) *Epistemology: A Contemporary Introduction to the 'Theory of Knowledge'* (London: Routledge).

Barnes J. (1982) *Aristotle* (Oxford: Oxford University Press).

Bauby J.-D. (1997) *The Diving Bell and the Butterfly* (London: Fourth Estate).

Benner P. (1984) *From Novice to Expert, Excellence and Power in Clinical Nursing Practice* (Menlo Park, CA: Addison-Wesley).

Benner P. (1985) 'Quality of life: a phenomenological perspective on explanation, prediction, and understanding in nursing science', *Advances in Nursing Science*, 8(1): 1–14.

Benner P. (ed.) (1994) *Interpretive Phenomenology* (London: Sage).

Benner P. (1994) 'The tradition and skill of interpretive phenomenology' in studying health, illness and caring practices' in *Interpretive Phenomenology: Embodiment, Caring and Ethics in Health and Illness*, P. Benner (ed.) (London: Sage) pp. 99–127.

Benner P. and Tanner C. (1987) 'How expert nurses use intuition', *American Journal of Nursing*, 87(1): 23–31.

Benner P. and Wrubel J. (1989) *The Primacy of Caring, Stress and Coping in Health and Illness* (Menlo Park, CA: Addison-Wesley).

Benner P., Tanner C. and Chesla C. (1996) *Expertise in Nursing Practice* (New York: Springer).

Berkeley G. ([1784]1972) *A New Theory of Vision, and Other Writings* (London: Everyman).

Bhaskar R. (1975) *A Realist Theory of Science* (Verso: London).

Bhaskar R. (1989) *The Possibility of Naturalism: A Philosophical Critique of the Contemporary Human Sciences*, 2nd edn (Hemel Hempstead: Harvester).

Bird G.H. (1972) *Philosophical Tasks* (London: RKP).

Bishop A.H. and Scudder J.R. (1991) *Nursing, the Practice of Caring* (New York: NLN Press).

Bishop A.H. and Scudder J.R. (1997) 'Nursing as a practice rather than an art or a science', *Nursing Outlook*, 45: 82–5.

Bishop A.H. and Scudder J.R. (1999) 'A philosophical interpretation of nursing', *Scholarly Inquiry in Nursing*, 13(1): 17–27.

Boorse C. (1975) 'On the distinction between disease and illness', *Philosophy and Public Affairs*, 5(1): 49–68.

Booth K., Kenrick M. and Woods S. (1997) 'Nursing knowledge, theory and method revisited', *Journal of Advanced Nursing*, 26: 804–11.

Brencick J.M. and Webster G.A. (2000) *Philosophy of Nursing, A New Vision for Health Care* (New York: State University of New York Press).

Burge T. (1979) 'Individualism and the mental' in *Midwest Studies in Philosophy*, 4: 73–121, P.A. French, T.E. Uehling and H.K. Wettstein (eds) (Minneapolis: University of Minnesota Press.)

Campbell K. (1984) *Body and Mind*, 2nd edn (Notre Dame, IN: University of Notre Dame Press).

Carper B.A. (1978) 'Fundamental patterns of knowing in nursing', *Advances in Nursing Science*, 1(1): 13–23.

Carruthers P. (1989) *Introducing Persons* (London: Routledge).

Cash K. (1990) 'Nursing models and the idea of nursing', *International Journal of Nursing Studies*, 27(3): 249–58.

Cash K. (1995) 'Benner and expertise in nursing: a critique', *International Journal of Nursing Studies*, 32(6): 527–34.

Cash K. (1998) 'Traditions and practice – nursing theory and political philosophy', in *Philosophical Issues in Nursing*, S.D. Edwards (ed.) (London: Macmillan – now Palgrave), pp. 31–46.

Cassell E.J. (1991) *The Nature of Suffering* (Oxford: Oxford University Press).

Chalmers A.F. (1982) *What is This Thing called Science?*, 2nd edn (Milton Keynes: Open University Press).

Chalmers A.F. (1990) *Science and Its Fabrication* (Milton Keynes: Open University Press).

Chalmers A.F. (1999) *What is This Thing called Science?*, 3rd edn (Milton Keynes: Open University Press).

Chinn P.L. and Kramer M.K. (1991) *Theory and Nursing: A Systematic Approach*, 3rd edn (St. Louis: Mosby).

Chinn P.L. and Watson J. (eds) (1994) *Art and Aesthetics in Nursing* (New York: NLN Press).

Churchland P.A. (1989) *Matter and Consciousness* (Cambridge, MA: MIT Press).

Clark J. (1999) 'The science of nursing', *Professional Nurse*, 13(9): 573.

Clarke L. (1999) 'The trouble with a specialised language for nursing', *Nursing Standard*, 14(2): 41–3.

Collingwood R.G. (1958) *The Principles of Art* (Oxford: Oxford University Press).

Comte A. ([1830]1970) *Introduction to Positive Philosophy* (Indianapolis: Bobbs-Merrill).

Davidson D. (1980) *Essays on Actions and Events* (Oxford: Oxford University Press).

De Raeve L. (1996) 'Caring intensively', in *Philosophical Problems in Health Care*, D. Greaves and H. Upton (eds) (Aldershot: Avebury), pp. 9–22.

De Raeve L. (1998) 'The art of nursing: an aesthetics?', *Nursing Ethics*, 5(5): 401–11.

Dennett D. (1981) *Brainstorms* (Brighton: Harvester Press).

Descartes R. (1954) *Philosophical Writings*, E. Anscombe and P. Geach (eds) (London: Open University Press).

Dickie G. (1971) *Aesthetics, An Introduction* (Indianapolis: Pegasus).

Dickoff J. and James P. (1968) 'A theory of theories: a position paper', *Nursing Research*, 17(3): 197–203.

Dillon M.C. (1997) *Merleau-Ponty's Ontology*, 2nd edn (Evanston, IL: Northwestern University Press).

Dreyfus H.L. (1991) *Being-in-the-World, A Commentary on Heidegger's Being and Time, Division 7* (Massachusetts: MIT Press).

Dreyfus H.L. (1994) 'Preface', in *Interpretive Phenomenology*, P. Benner (ed.) (London: Sage), pp. vii–xi.

Dreyfus S.E. and Dreyfus H.L. (1980) *A Five-stage Model of the Mental Activities involved in Directed Skill Acquisition* (Berkeley, CA: University of California/USAF).

Dunlop M.J. (1986) 'Is a science of caring possible?', *Journal of Advanced Nursing*, 11: 661–70.

Dunne J. (1993) *Back to the Rough Ground, Practical Judgment and the Lure of Technique* (Notre Dame, IN: University of Notre Dame Press).

Edwards S.D. (1990) *Relativism, Conceptual Schemes and Categorial Frameworks* (Aldershot: Avebury).

Edwards S.D. (1994) *Externalism in the Philosophy of Mind* (Aldershot: Avebury).

Edwards S.D. (1996) *Nursing Ethics: A Principle-Based Approach* (London: Macmillan – now Palgrave).

Edwards S.D (1997) 'What is philosophy of nursing?', *Journal of Advanced Nursing*, 25: 1089–93.

Edwards S.D. (ed.) (1998a) *Philosophical Issues in Nursing* (London: Macmillan – now Palgrave).

Edwards S.D. (1998b) 'The art of nursing', *Nursing Ethics*, 5(5): 393–400.

English I. (1993) 'Intuition as a function of the expert nurse, a critique of Benner's novice to expert model', *Journal of Advanced Nursing*, 18: 387–93.

Fawcett J. (1995) *Analysis and Evaluation of Conceptual Models of Nursing*, 3rd edn (Philadelphia: Davis).

Fay B. (1996) *Contemporary Philosophy of Social Science* (Oxford: Blackwell).

Ferguson A. (1999) *Managing My Life* (London: Hodder & Stoughton).

Fiser K.B. (1986) 'Privacy and pain', *Philosophical Investigations*, 9(1): 1–17.

Flew A. (1979) *Dictionary of Philosophy* (London: Pan Books).

Fodor J. (1983) *The Modularity of Mind* (Cambridge, MA: MIT Press).

Fry S.T. (1989) 'Toward a theory of nursing ethics', *Advances in Nursing Science*, 11(3): 9–22.

Gadow S. (1982) 'Body and self', in *The Humanity of the Ill, Phenomenological Perspectives*, V. Kestenbaum (ed.) (Knoxville: University of Tennessee Press), pp. 86–100.

Gadow S. (1989) 'Clinical subjectivity, advocacy with silent patients', *Nursing Clinics of North America*, 24(2): 535–41.

Gadow S. (1995) 'Clinical epistemology: a dialectic of nursing assessment', *Canadian Journal of Nursing Research*, 27(2): 35–44.

Gardner S. (1995) 'Aesthetics' in *Philosophy, A Guide Through the Subject*, A.C. Grayling (ed.) (Oxford: Oxford University Press), pp. 585–627.

Gettier E. (1963) 'Is justified true belief knowledge?', *Analysis*, 23: 121–3.

Gortner S.R. (1990) 'Nursing values and science: toward a science philosophy', *Image*, 22(2): 101–5.

Grayling A.C. (1995) *Philosophy, A Guide Through the Subject* (Oxford: Oxford University Press).

Greaves D. (1996) 'Concepts of health, illness and disease' in *Philosophical Problems in Health Care*, D. Greaves and H. Upton (eds) (Aldershot: Avebury), pp. 71–86.

Greenhalgh T. and Hurwitz B. (eds) (1998) *Narrative-based Medicine* (London: BMJ).

Gross R.D. (1987) *Psychology, The Science of Mind and Behaviour* (London: Hodder & Stoughton).

Haber R.N. and Hershenson M. (1980) *The Psychology of Visual Perception* (New York: Holt, Rinehart & Winston).

Halfpenny P. (1982) *Positivism and Sociology* (London: George Allen & Unwin).

Hall H. (1983) 'Merleau-Ponty's philosophy of mind', in *Contemporary Philosophy, A New Survey*, G. Floistad (ed.) (The Hague: Nijhoff) 4: 343–61.

Hamlyn D.W. (1970) *The Theory of Knowledge* (London: Macmillan – now Palgrave).

Hammond M., Howarth J. and Keat R. (1991) *Understanding Phenomenology* (Oxford: Blackwell).

Hanfling O. (ed.) (1992) *Philosophical Aesthetics, An Introduction* (Oxford: Oxford University Press).

Harris J. (1985) *The Value of Life* (London: RKP).

Hegel G.W.F. (1894) *Hegel's Philosophy of Mind*, W. Wallace (trans.) (Oxford: Clarendon Press).

Heidegger M. (1962) *Being and Time*, J. Macquarrie and E. Robinson (trans.) (Oxford: Blackwell).

Hempel C.G. (1966) *Philosophy of Natural Science* (Englewood Cliffs, NJ: Prentice-Hall).

Henderson V. (1966) *The Nature of Nursing: A Definition and Its Implications for Practice, Education and Research* (London: Macmillan – now Palgrave).

Hiley D.R., Bohman J.F. and Shusterman R. (eds) (1991) *The Interpretive Turn* (Ithaca, NY: Cornell University Press).

Holden R.J. (1991) 'In defence of Cartesian dualism and the hermeneutic horizon', *Journal of Advanced Nursing*, 16: 1375–81.

Honderich T. (ed.) (1992) *The Oxford Companion to Philosophy* (Oxford: Oxford University Press).

Husserl E. (1931) *Ideas* (New York: Collier Books).

Hussey T. (2000) 'Realism and Nursing', *Nursing Philosophy*, 1(2): 98–108.

Johns C. (1995) 'Framing learning through reflection within Carper's fundamental ways of knowing in nursing', *Journal of Advanced Nursing*, 22(2): 226–34.

Johnson J.L. (1994) 'A dialectical examination of nursing art', *Advances in Nursing Science*, 17(1): 1–14.

Kerby A.P. (1991) *Narrative and the Self* (Indianapolis: Indiana University Press).

Kikuchi J.F. and Simmons H. (eds) (1992) *Philosophic Inquiry in Nursing* (London: Sage).

Kikuchi J.F. and Simmons H. (eds) (1994) *Developing a Philosophy of Nursing* (London: Sage).

Kikuchi J.F. and Simmons H. (1996) 'The whole truth, and progress in nursing knowledge development', in *Truth in Nursing Inquiry*, J.F. Kikuchi, H. Simmons and D. Romyn (eds) (London: Sage), pp. 5–18.

Kikuchi J.F., Simmons H. and Romyn D. (eds) (1996) *Truth in Nursing Inquiry*, (London: Sage).

Kim J. (1995) 'Explanatory exclusion and the problem of mental causation' in *Philosophy of Psychology*, C. Macdonald and G. Macdonald (eds) (Oxford: Blackwell), pp. 121–41.

King I. and Fawcett J. (eds) (1997) *The Language of Nursing Theory and Metatheory* (Indianapolis: Center Nursing Press).

Kitwood T. (1997) *Dementia Reconsidered* (Milton Keynes: Open University Press).

Kleinman A. (1986) *Social Origins of Distress and Disease: Depression, Neurasthenia and Pain in Modern China* (New Haven, CT: Yale University Press).

Kleinman A. (1988) *Illness Narratives: Suffering, Healing and the Human Condition* (New York: Basic Books).

Kripke S. (1972) *Naming and Necessity* (Oxford: Blackwell).

Kuhn T.S. (1970) *The Structure of Scientific Revolutions*, 2nd edn (Chicago: University of Chicago Press).

Kuhse H. (1997) *Caring: Nurses, Women and Ethics* (Oxford: Oxford University Press).

Langer M.M. (1989) *Merleau-Ponty's 'Phenomenology of Perception', A Guide and Commentary* (London: Macmillan – now Palgrave).

Leininger M.M. (ed.) (1984) *Care: The Essence of Nursing and Health* (New York: Slack).

Liaschenko J. (1998) 'The shift from the closed to the open body...', in *Philosophical Issues in Nursing*, S.D. Edwards (ed.) (London: Macmillan – now Palgrave), pp. 11–30.

Liaschenko J. and Davis A.J. (1991) 'Nurses and physicians on nutritional support: a comparison', *Journal of Medicine and Philosophy*, 16: 259–83.

Luper-Foy S. (1992) 'Knowledge and belief', in *A Companion to Epistemology*, J. Dancy and E. Sosa (eds) (Oxford: Oxford University Press), pp. 234–7.

Macdonald C. (1989) *Mind–Body Identity Theories* (London: Routledge).

Macdonald C. (1990) 'Weak externalism and mind–body identity', *Mind*, 99: 387–405.

Macdonald C. and Macdonald G. (eds) (1995) *Philosophy of Psychology* (Oxford: Blackwell).

McGinn C. (1982) *The Character of Mind* (Oxford: Oxford University Press).

McGinn C. (1998) *The Character of Mind*, 2nd edn (Oxford: Oxford University Press).

MacIntyre A. (1983) 'To whom is the nurse responsible?', in *Ethical Problems in the Nurse–Patient Relationship*, C.D. Murphy and H. Hunter (eds) (Boston: Allyn & Bacon), pp. 79–83.

MacIntyre A. (1985) *After Virtue* (London: Duckworth).

MacIntyre A. (1999) *Dependent Rational Animals* (London: Duckworth).

McKenna H. (1997) *Nursing Theories and Models* (London: Routledge).

Malmsten K. (1999) *Reflective Assent in Basic Care* (Uppsala: Uppsala University Press).

Marriner-Tomey A. (1994) *Nursing Theorists and Their Work*, 3rd edn (St Louis: Mosby).

Mayerhoff M. (1971) *On Caring* (New York: Harper & Row).

Meleis A.I. (1985) *Theoretical Nursing: Development and Progress* (Philadelphia: Lippincott).

Merleau-Ponty M. (1962) *The Phenomenology of Perception*, (trans.) C. Smith (London: Routledge).

Merleau-Ponty M. (1968) *The Visible and the Invisible*, (ed.) C. Lefort (Evanston, IL: Northwestern University Press).

Merrell S.B. (1998) *Defining Personhood: Toward the Ethics of Quality in Clinical Care* (Amsterdam: Rodopi).

Morris J. (1991) *Pride Against Prejudice* (London: Women's Press).

Moser P.K. (1992) 'Tripartite definition of knowledge', in *Companion to Epistemology*, J. Dancy and E. Sosa (eds) (Oxford: Oxford University Press), p. 509.

Mulhall S. (1996) *Heidegger and Being and Time* (London: Routledge).

Nagel T. (1987) *What Does it All Mean? A Very Short Introduction to Philosophy* (Oxford: Oxford University Press).

Newton-Smith W.H. (1981) *The Rationality of Science* (London: RKP).

Nightingale F. (1957/1859) *Notes on Nursing* (Philadelphia: Lippincott).

Noddings N. (1984) *Caring: A Feminine Approach to Ethics and Moral Education* (Berkeley, CA: University of California Press).

Nordenfelt L. (1993) 'On the notions of disability and handicap', *Social Welfare*, 2: 17–24.

Nordenfelt L. (1995) *On the Nature of Health, An Action–Theoretic Approach*, 2nd edn (Dordrecht: Kluwer).

Nortvedt P. (1996) *Sensitive Judgement, Nursing, Moral Philosophy and an Ethics of Care* (Sats Norway: Tano Aschehoug).

Nortvedt P. (1998) 'Sensitive judgement: an inquiry into the foundations of nursing ethics', *Nursing Ethics*, 5(5): 385–92.

O'Hear A. (1989) *An Introduction to the Philosophy of Science* (Oxford: Oxford University Press).

Orem D.E. (1971) *Nursing Concepts of Practice* (New York: McGraw-Hill).

Orem D.E. (1987) 'Orem's general theory of nursing', in *Nursing Science, Major Paradigms, Theories and Critiques* R.R. Parse (ed.) (London: W.B. Saunders) pp. 67–89.

Paley J. (1996) 'Intuition and expertise: comments on the Benner debate', *Journal of Advanced Nursing*, **23**: 665–71.

Paley J. (1997) 'Husserl, phenomenology and nursing', *Journal of Advanced Nursing*, **26**: 87–93.

Paley J. (1999) 'Body, mind, expertise: notes on the polarisation of health care discourse', in *Social Policy and the Body: Transitions in Corporeal Discourses* H. Dean and K. Ellis (eds) (London: Macmillan – now Palgrave), pp. 103–21.

Paley J. (2000) 'Heidegger and the ethics of care', *Nursing Philosophy*, **1**: 64–75.

Parfit D. (1986) *Reasons and Persons* (Oxford. Clarendon Press).

Parse R.R. (1981) *Man–Living–Health, A Theory of Nursing* (New York: Wiley).

Parse R.R. (ed.) (1987) *Nursing Science, Major Paradigms, Theories and Critiques* (London: W.B. Saunders).

Parse R.R. (1995) 'Building the realm of nursing knowledge', *Nursing Science Quarterly*, **8**: 51. (New York: NLN Press).

Parse R.R. (1998) *The Human Becoming School of Thought* (London: Sage).

Peplau H.E. (1987) 'Nursing science: a historical perspective', in *Nursing Science: Major Paradigms, Theories and Critiques* R.R. Parse (ed.) (London: W.B. Saunders), pp. 13–29.

Plato *The Republic* (trans.) D. Lee (1974) (London: Penguin).

Plato *Theaetetus* (trans.) F.M. Cornford (1957) (Indianapolis: Bobbs-Merrill).

Polanyi M. (1958) *Personal Knowledge* (London: Routledge & Kegan Paul).

Polifroni E.C. and Welch M. (eds) (1999) *Perspectives on Philosophy of Science in Nursing* (New York: Lippincott).

Popkin R.H. and Stroll A. (1993) *Philosophy Made Simple*, 3rd edn (London: Butterworth-Heinemann).

Popper K. (1963) *Conjectures and Refutations* (London: RKP).

Priest S. (1998) *Merleau-Ponty* (London: Routledge).

Quine W.V.O. (1951) 'Two dogmas of empiricism', in *Philosophical Review*, **60**: 20–43, reprinted in *From a Logical Point of View* W.V.O. Quine (ed.) (1961) (Cambridge, MA: Harvard University Press), pp. 20–46.

Quine W.V.O. and Ullian J.S. (1978) *The Web of Belief* (New York: Random House).

Quinn E.V. and Prest J.M. (eds) (1987) *Dear Miss Nightingale, A Selection of Benjamin Jowett's Letters 1860–1893* (Oxford: Clarendon Press).

Quinton A. (1995) 'Philosophy', in *The Oxford Companion to Philosophy* T. Honderich (ed.) (Oxford: Oxford University Press), pp. 666–70.

Reed J. and Ground I. (1997) *Philosophy for Nursing* (London: Arnold).

Revans R.W. (1964) *Cause and Effect in Hospitals* (London: published for the Nuffield Provincial Hospitals Trust by Oxford University Press).

Ricoeur P. (1992) *Oneself as Another* (Chicago: University of Chicago Press).

Robinson K. and Vaughan B. (eds) (1992) *Knowledge for Nursing Practice* (Oxford: Butterworth-Heinemann).

Rodgers B.L. (1991) 'Deconstructing the dogma in nursing knowledge and practice', *Image*, **23**(3): 177–81.

Rogers M.E. (1970) *An Introduction to the Theoretical Basis of Nursing* (Philadelphia: F.A. Davis & Co.).

Rogers M.E. (1987) 'Rogers' science of unitary human beings' in *Nursing Science, Major Paradigms, Theories and Critiques* R.R. Parse (ed.), (London: W.B. Saunders) pp. 139–46.

Rorty R. (1989) *Contingency, Irony, Solidarity* (Cambridge: Cambridge University Press).

Roy C. (1976) *Introduction to Nursing: An Adaptation Model* (Englewood Cliffs, NJ: Prentice-Hall).

Roy C. (1980) 'The Roy adaptation model' in *Conceptual Models for Nursing Practice* J.P Riehl and C. Roy (eds) (New York: Appleton-Century-Crofts), pp. 179–88.

Roy C. (1987) 'Roy's adaptation model' in *Nursing Science, Major Paradigms, Theories and Critiques* R.R. Parse (ed.) (London: W.B. Saunders), pp. 35–46.

Russell B. (1912) *The Problems of Philosophy* (Oxford: Oxford University Press).

Russell B. (1939) *A History of Western Philosophy* (London: Allen & Unwin).

Ryle G. (1949) *The Concept of Mind* (Harmondsworth: Penguin).

Sacks O. (1984) *A Leg to Stand On* (London: Picador).

Schectman M (1996) *The Constitution of Selves* (New York: Cornell University Press).

Schultz P.R. and Meleis A.I. (1988) 'Nursing epistemology: traditions, insights, questions', *Image*, **20**(4): 217–21.

Schröck R. (1981a) 'Philosophical issues', in *Current Issues in Nursing* L. Hockey (ed.) (Edinburgh: Churchill Livingstone), pp. 3–18.

Schröck R. (1981b) 'Philosophical perspectives', in *Nursing Science in Nursing Practice* J.P. Smith (ed.) (London: Butterworths), pp. 170–84.

Schumacher K.L. and Gortner S.R. (1992) '(Mis)conceptions and reconceptions about traditional science', *Advances in Nursing Science*, **14**(4): 1–11.

Scott A.P. (2000) 'Emotion, moral perception, and nursing practice', *Nursing Philosophy*, **1**(2): pp. 123–33.

Sellman D. (2000) 'Alasdair MacIntyre and the professional practice of nursing', *Nursing Philosophy*, **1**(1): 26–33.

Shusterman R. (1991) 'Beneath interpretation' in *The Interpretive Turn* D.R. Hiley, J.F. Bohman and R. Shusterman (eds) (Ithaca, NY: Cornell University Press), pp. 102–28.

Silva M.C. and Rothbart D. (1984) 'An analysis of changing trends in philosophies of science on nursing theory development and testing', *Advances in Nursing Science*, **6**(2): 1–13.

Singer P. (1990) *Animal Liberation*, 2nd edn (New York: Random House).

Smith N.H. (1997) *Strong Hermeneutics* (London: Routledge).

Spicker S.F. and Gadow S. (1980) *Nursing: Images and Ideals* (New York: Springer).

Szasz T.S. (1972) *The Myth of Mental Illness* (London: Paladin).

Taylor C. (1985) 'Self-interpreting animals', in *Philosophical Papers*, Vol. 1 C. Taylor (ed.) (Cambridge: Cambridge University Press), pp. 45–76.

Thagard P. (1998) 'Ulcers and bacteria I, discovery and acceptance', *Studies in History, Biology and Biomedical Science*, **29**(1): 107–36.

Toombs S.K. (1993) *The Meaning of Illness* (Dordrecht: Kluwer).

Toombs S.K. (1995) 'Sufficient unto the day: a life with multiple sclerosis', in *Chronic Illness, From Experience to Policy* S.K. Toombs, D. Barnard and R.A. Carson (eds) (Indianapolis: Indiana University Press), pp. 3–33.

Upton H.R. (1998) 'Can philosophy legitimately be applied?' in *Critical Reflection on Medical Ethics* M. Evans (ed.) (London: JAI Press), pp. 123–38.

van Hooft S. (1987) 'Caring and professional commitment', *Australian Journal of Advanced Nursing*, **4**(4): 29–38.

van Hooft S. (1995) *Caring, An Essay in the Philosophy of Ethics* (Boulder: University Press of Colorado).

van Os J., Galdos P., Lewis G., Bourgeois M. and Mann A. (1993) 'Schizophrenia sans frontieres: concepts of schizophrenia among French and British psychiatrists', *British Medical Journal*, **307**: 489–92.

Wainwright P. (1997) 'The practice of nursing: an investigation of professional nursing from the perspective of the virtue ethics of Alasdair MacIntyre', unpublished PhD thesis, University of Wales, Swansea.

Wainwright P. (1999) 'The art of nursing', *International Journal of Nursing Studies*, **36**: 379–85.

Wainwright S. (1997) 'A new paradigm for nursing, the potential of realism', *Journal of Advanced Nursing*, **26**: 1262–71.

Warner R. and Szubka T. (eds) (1994) *The Mind–Body Problem: A Guide to the Current Debate* (Oxford: Blackwell).

Wartofsky M. (1992) 'The social presuppositions of medical knowledge' in J.L. Peset and D. Gracia (eds) *The Ethics of Diagnosis* (Dordrecht: Kluwer), pp. 131–51.

Watson J. (1979) *Nursing: The Philosophy and Science of Caring* (Boulder: University Press of Colorado).

Watson J. (1988) *Nursing: Human Science and Human Care* (New York: NLN Press).

Watson J.D. (1968) *The Double Helix: A Personal Account of the Discovery of the Structure of DNA* (London: Weidenfeld & Nicolson).

Wilson E. (1979) *The Mental as Physical* (London: RKP).

Wittgenstein L. (1953) *Philosophical Investigations* (Oxford: Blackwell).

Wittgenstein L. (1975) *On Certainty* (Oxford, Blackwell).

Wulff H.R. (1994) 'The disease concept and the medical view of man', in *The Discipline of Medicine* A.Querida, L.A. von Es and E. Mademe (eds) (Dordrecht: Kluwer).

Wulff H.R., Pederson S.A. and Rosenberg R. (1986) *Philosophy of Medicine, An Introduction* (Oxford: Blackwell).

Index

A

Ackrill, J.L. 199
Advances in Nursing Science 4, 136
aesthetics 10, 11, 44
Aggleton, P. and Chalmers, H. 72
Alston, W.P. 48
appeals to authority 6, 31, 65
Aristotle 6, 20, 53, 137–8, 158, 198, 199
Armstrong, D.M. 72
art of nursing 41, 78, 157–63
    art/craft distinction 157–63
art, theories of 158
Asimov, I. 61
Audi, R. 66

B

basic care 63–4
Bauby, J-D. 81
Beckham, D. 128–9
Benner, P. 1, 3, 4, 9, 14, 19, 21, 23, 31, 38, 39, 40, 49–60, 64, 65, 66, 95, 143, 148–9, 150, 153, 155, 164, 165, 166, 170, 178, 181, 184, 188, 192
    From Novice to Expert (FNE) 49–60
Benner, P. and Tanner, C. 59
Benner, P. and Wrubel, J. 4, 17, 32, 34, 35, 67, 69, 70, 77, 78, 81, 82, 83, 90, 97, 98, 105, 110, 124–30, 145, 146, 147, 165, 183, 185, 187, 190, 193
Berkeley, G. 6
Bhaskar, R. 142, 145, 147, 150–6, 174, 176
Bird, G. 7

Bishop, A.H. and Scudder, J.R. 4, 5, 20, 114, 138, 140, 141, 158, 163, 167–8, 169, 170, 171, 174
bodily intentionality 34–5, 55
Boorse, C. 72
Booth, K. 27, 28
Brencick, J.M. and Webster, G.A. 20
Burge, T. 148

C

Carper, B.A. 1, 4, 11, 14, 15, 16, 21, 23, 38, 39, 40–9, 60, 64, 'Fundamental patterns of knowing in nursing' (FPKN) 23, 40–9, 157
    on empirics 40, 41, 43, 47,
    on 'esthetics' 40, 41, 44–5, 47, 48
    on personal knowing 40, 42, 45, 48, 49
    on ethical knowing 40, 42, 46, 48, 49
Campbell, K. 107
care and caring 109–34, 163
    deep care 124, 128–30, 193
    ethical caring 117–18
    identity-constituting care 124, 128–30, 132, 134, 140, 193
    intentional care 109–23, 125, 127, 131–4, 193
    natural caring 117–18
    ontological care 110, 124–35, 193
    reciprocal 116–17, 118
Carruthers, P. 107
Cartesian dualism 67, 77, 78, 81, 82, 83, 85, 105, 192

Cash, K. ix, 5, 8, 52, 56, 57, 172, 173, 189–90
Cassell, E.J. 75, 77, 95
Chalmers, A.F. 143, 174, 176, 191
Chinn, P.L. and Kramer, M.K. 22, 23
Chinn, P.L. and Watson, J. 157, 174
Clark, J. 136
Clarke, L. 136
Collingwood, R.G. 157–63, 174
Comte, A. 142
conservatism (as a virtue) 28, 57, 84, 192
conservatism (as a criticism of Benner) 56–8
Copernicus, N. 27

D

dancer example 69, 94, 104, 106
Dasein 125, 126, 130
Davidson, D. 110
Davis, A. 63
dementia 99–100
Dennett, D. 87
dependence/reduction distinction 67, 75, 82, 85–6, 105
de Raeve, L. ix, 44, 100, 121, 133, 174
Descartes, R. 20, 27, 77
descriptive/evaluative distinction 139, 179
Dickie, G. 174
Dickoff, J. and James, P. 4, 8, 175, 177–81, 186, 189, 191
Dillon, M.C. 83, 108
Dreyfus, H.L. 32
Dreyfus, S.E. and Dreyfus, H.L. 4, 50
Dunlop, M. 148

E

Edwards, S.D. 5, 16, 83, 198
Einstein, A. 27
emotion 119–21, 132, 162
emotional understanding 119
English, I. 52, 59

entailment thesis 37
epistemology 9, 195
ethics 10, 11
Evans, H.M. ix

F

Fawcett, J. 4, 62
Fay, B. 108, 174
Ferguson, A. 92
Fiser, K.B. 74
Flew, A. 13–14, 195
Fodor, J. 79
foetus, the 101–2
Freud, S. 45
Fry, S. 114

G

Gadow, S. 4, 5, 19, 80–1, 147, 183–4
Gardner, S. 158, 174
generalisations 181–5, 187
Gettier, E. 26, 27
Gortner, S. 4, 143
Grayling, A.C. 19, 66, 107
Greaves, D. ix, 68, 72
Greenhalgh, T. and Hurwitz, B. 97
Gross, R.D. 73
Ground, I. 4

H

Haber, R.N. and Hershenson, M. 53
Halfpenny, P. 142, 144
Hall, H. 79
Hamlyn, D.W. 36, 37, 66
Hammond, M. 34, 108
Hanfling, O. 174
Harris, J. 101
health 68, 95, 106, 179
   biostatistical view 68–9
   holistic view 68–9
health promotion 97–9
Heath, E. 88
Hegel, G.W.F. 4
Heidegger, M. 4, 17, 32, 53, 119, 120, 125, 126, 127, 130, 135, 198

Hempel, C. 145, 191, 199
Henderson, V. 3, 70
hermeneutic universalism 147
Hiley, D.R. 145
Holden, R. 70, 77, 78, 85
Honderich, T. 195
Hume, D. 20
Husserl, E. 17, 196
Hussey, T. 148, 150

I

ideological intoxication 147
Image 4
Ince, P. 92
Institute for Philosophical Research
    in Nursing 4
intellectualist model (of practical
    knowledge) 33, 34, 35
internal goods 165–8, 171
    distinct from external goods 165
interpretivism 145–50, 153, 155
    and realism 149–50
intuition 52–3, 58–60
    as mysticism 52–3, 58–9
invisible knowledge 186

J

Johns, C. 40
Johnson, J. 157, 159
Journal of Advanced Nursing 4
Journal of Applied Philosophy 18
Jowett, B. 3

K

Kant, I. 20
Kerby, A.P. 91, 101, 108
Kikuchi, J. 4, 21
Kikuchi, J. and Simmons, H. 5, 20,
    25
Kim, J. 76
King, I. 4, 175
King, I. and Fawcett, J. 175, 191
Kitwood, T. 99
Kleinman, A. 96, 97

knowledge/belief distinction 24–6,
    43
    within practical knowledge 38,
        54
Kripke, S. 74
Kuhn, T.S. 146
Kuhse, H. 63

L

Langer, M 108
Leininger, M. 109, 126
Liaschenko, J. 63, 186, 188
logic 11
Luper-Foy, S. 37

M

Macdonald, C. 83
Macdonald, C. and Macdonald, G.
    76
MacIntyre, A. 4, 88, 90, 96,
    164–71, 173, 174, 194
Malmsten, K. 63–4
Marriner-Tomey, A. 3, 5, 22
Maxwell, R. 92
McGinn, C. 76, 83, 107
McKenna, H. 22, 40, 41, 70, 191
medical knowledge 62
medical model 72
Melies, A.I. 4
Merleau-Ponty, M. 4, 17, 34, 36,
    51, 67, 70, 78–84, 85, 96, 87, 88,
    105, 192, 196
Merrell, S.B. 198
Mill, J.S. 3
mind–body problem 71–2, 192
mini-narratives 89–90, 92
modesty 29, 65, 67, 84, 134, 170,
    181, 192
Moore, D. ix
moral phenomenology 11
moral pull 117, 118, 123, 133, 134
Morris, R. 98
Moser, P.K. 26
Mulhall, S. 125, 135, 146
Muller-Lyer illusion 47

N

Nagel, T. 19, 66, 107
narrative understanding 91, 92–3, 94, 95, 96–102, 105, 140, 173, 180, 182, 183, 184–5, 190, 192
necessary and contingent truths distinction 12–13, 24, 48, 73–4, 102–3
necessary and sufficient conditions distinction 13–14, 87
Newton, I. 27
Newton-Smith, W. 27, 29
Nightingale, F. 3, 62, 103, 157
Noddings, N. 109, 110, 114–19, 121
Nordenfelt, L. 95, 190
Nortvedt, P. 95, 119, 120, 131, 132, 135, 189
novice/expert distinction 49–55, 56–7
N-states 73, 74
nursing as a practice 164–74, 175, 190, 194
nursing ethics 5, 11
Nursing Ethics 5
nursing knowledge Chs. 2–3 *passim*, esp. 60–6
Nursing Philosophy 5
Nursing-philosophy@mailbase.ac.uk 5
Nursing Science Quarterly 136

O

O'Hear, A. 136
ontological depth 151–2, 154
ontology 10
Orem, D. 4, 5, 63, 69, 136, 189

P

Paley, J. ix, 5, 17, 56, 130, 135, 148
Parfit, D. 87
Parse, R.R. 4, 22, 61, 62, 63, 64, 67, 70, 78, 97, 136, 191
Peplau, H.E. 136
persistent vegetative state (PVS) 100–1, 102, 114, 121–2, 191, 192–3

phenomenology 80–1, 196
philosophical inquiry 6–14
    first- and second-order questions in 7–8
philosophy of medicine 2
philosophy of nursing 14–19, 171
    defined 14
    its location within philosophy 18 19
    philosophical presuppositions strand 15–16, 40
    philosophical problems strand 15–16
    scholarship strand 16–17, 22, 40
Plato 20, 26, 32, 158
plight 102, 112, 116, 117, 120, 122, 123, 131, 132, 134, 191
Polanyi, M. 53
Polifroni, E.C. and Welch, M. 174
Popkin, R.H. and Stroll, A. 20, 66, 107
Popper, K. 30
positivism 142–5, 155
practical belief 38
practical knowledge 31–9, 41–2, 53–6, 186, 187, 188, 192
pre-operative fasting 28, 29, 30
Priest, S. 81, 108
principle of postural echo 50, 51, 182, 187, 188, 189
propositional knowledge 21–31, 32, 53–6, 186, 187, 188, 192
P-states 73, 74
Ptolemy 27

Q

quality of life 95, 106, 153, 154, 179
Quine, W.V.O. 21, 27, 28, 31, 43, 104, 197
Quine, W.V.O. and Ullian, J.S. 27, 28, 29, 30, 31, 57, 59, 66, 67, 86, 149, 174, 176, 192
    and virtues of hypotheses and beliefs 28–31, 67, 149
Quinn, E.V. and Prest, J.M. 3
Quinton, A. 7

R

realism   149, 150–6
Reed, J.   4
Reed, J. and Ground, I.   5, 16, 20
Revans, R.W.   185
refutability   30
Ricoeur, P.   91, 108
Robinson, K. and Vaughan, B.   21
Rodgers, B.   31, 65
Rogers, M.   4, 5
Romyn, D.   20
Rorty, R.   104
Roy, C.   4, 5, 70
Russell, B.   6, 7
Ryle, G.   21, 32, 33, 35, 53, 66, 186

S

Sacks, O.   36, 37
salience   51–2
scepticism   27
Schectman, M.   108
Schröck, R.   4
Schumacher, K.L. and Gortner, S.R.
     143, 148, 150
Scott, P.A.   119, 189
Scudder, J.R.   4
self-conception   1, 89, 91, 185, 190
self-project   1, 89, 91, 93, 95, 96,
     102, 134, 135, 180, 182, 183,
     185, 192
Sellman, D.   163, 173, 174
Shoemaker, S. and Swinburne, R.
     87
Shusterman, R.   147
Silva, M.C.   4
Silva, M.C. and Rothbart, D.   4
Simmons, H.   4
simplicity   29
situation producing theories   177–8
Smith, N.   13, 104
Spicker, S.   4
structuring concepts   94
sudden infant death syndrome   27
suffering   95, 106, 112, 123, 153,
     154, 162, 179
supervenience   76

survey list   178
sympathic awareness   131
Szasz, T.S.   57

T

Taylor, C.   4, 90, 91, 119
Thagard, P.   151
Thatcher, M.   88, 103
token identity   75, 76, 82, 105
Toombs, S.K.   98
tripartite criterion of knowledge   26,
     27
type identity   72, 84, 105

U

uniqueness claim   109
unity requirement   2, 175, 190, 194
University of Brighton   4
University of Wales Swansea   4
Upton, H.R.   18
uterus example   54, 55

V

value enquiry   10
van Hooft, S.   89, 113, 119, 120,
     127, 128, 135
van Os, J.   57
violent episodes example   44, 56, 65
vulnerability   111–12, 123, 193

W

Wainwright, P.   ix, 44, 163, 173, 174
Wainwright, S.   148, 150, 156
Warner, R. and Szubka, T.   107
Wartofsky, M.   62, 63
Watson, James   29
Watson, Jean   4, 20, 70, 77, 78, 85,
     109, 113, 114, 126, 157
Weidenbach, E.   3
Wilson, E.   72
Wittgenstein, L.   36, 37, 147, 148,
     189
Wulff, H.   185, 191